Praise for *Finding Me In Menopause*

'Dr Bajekal emphasises the importance of underpinning any recommended medical interventions such as HRT with appropriate advice about diet, lifestyle, exercise and so on. These key "basics" form the template to optimise menopause quality of life and long-term wellbeing for both the individual and society.'

Professor Nick Panay FRCOG, Consultant Gynaecologist with a special interest in Menopause

'Indispensable, engaging and evidence-based.'

Dr Rupy Aujla, 'The Doctor's Kitchen'

'The world needs this book! Dr Nitu provides such practical evidence-based advice from decades of experience to help women through menopause.'

The Happy Pear

'A brilliant insight to perimenopause and menopause from a doctor who has gone the extra mile to help women. Dr Nitu Bajekal's much needed book shares her own experiences, along with all her knowledge and research from decades of working in women's health.'

Suzi Shaw, singer/actress, and wellness advocate

'This book will become required reading for every woman. Empowering and compassionate, Nitu provides a whole health approach to supporting both physical and mental wellbeing. The knowledge acquired will help you to personalize your own decisions around the menopause whilst being reassured you are using an evidence-based source. A must read.'

Dr Shireen Kassam, Consultant Haematologist and Founder of Plant-Based Health Professionals UK

'As a gynaecological oncologist, I often have to induce an early menopause by surgically removing ovaries for gynaecological cancers. In some women, the fear of menopause is greater than the fear of cancer. Social media abounds with myths about the menopause and in particular, there is a suggestion that all the unpleasant symptoms are inevitable. This book is timely and informative. It empowers women to take charge of their menopause by providing evidence-based options; I will certainly encourage patients, colleagues, friends and relatives to read it.'

Miss Adeola Olaitan, FRCOG Consultant ObGyn

'A must-read for anyone embarking on the journey of perimenopause and menopause. Dr Nitu's heartfelt account and expert guidance provide the essential guide to navigating this phase of life with confidence and grace.'

Dr Alan Desmond, Consultant Gastroenterologist

'*Finding Me in Menopause* is a great book! It explains so much about the menopause and perimenopause and breaks things down in an easy to digest format. Tells you what you need to know! Well-researched, but not too scientific. This is not a preachy book, more like receiving great advice from a best friend (but with the knowledge and expertise to back it up). I highly recommend it to anyone looking for more than just a book - it's a journey towards positive change.'

Ayse Gul, Naturopathic Nutritional Therapist and Herbalist

'Scientifically factual yet jargon-free, this book has allowed me to take control of my menopause journey and has taught me so much about my own body and how to look after myself. The Menopause Mantras at the end of each chapter break everything down into positive achievable goals allowing you to take what you want from this book and incorporate it into your life and whatever level you feel comfortable with. Reading this is like sharing a coffee and a chat with a good friend who is there to help you every step of the way.'

Michelle, patient advocate

'A powerful manifesto of the power of holistic and lifestyle medicine in managing menopause. Dr Bakejal writes with empathy and kindness, but carefully balances this with deep knowledge and expertise. Her tone is reassuring, and by sharing her own story and personal journey with menopause, the book becomes really relatable. I enjoyed this book – especially the case studies at the end – and as a doctor and innovator within women's health, I will be recommending it to our customers and community.'

Dr Dupe Burgess, Founder and CEO, Bloomful

'I am so grateful that Dr Bajekal has written this incredible lifestyle-medicine based resource! Not only has it helped answer many questions about my own journey into perimenopause, it has also helped inform me on what is to come and what steps I can take to better take care of myself during this transition. I am eager to share this empowering knowledge with my coaching clients. Thank you, Dr Nitu Bajekal for this invaluable resource!'

Dr Yami Cazorla-Lancaster, Author of *A Parent's Guide to Intuitive Eating: How to Raise Kids Who Love to Eat Healthy*

'A transformative book... the ultimate guide to navigating menopause. Dr Nitu reframes the perimenopause and menopause experience.'

Dr Gemma Newman MBBCH DRCOG DFSRH MRCGP, GP and author

'A truly inspiring, educational and practical read... Dr Nitu breaks things down to simple, understandable terms and offers practical and simple everyday advice to help manage menopause.'

Lucy, patient advocate

'*Finding Me in Menopause* is the book I wish I'd had ten years ago. With warmth and compassion, and remaining inclusive throughout, Dr Bajekal brings together the latest evidence-based research in lifestyle medicine and applies it to the menopausal transition in a practical, non-judgemental, way. I will be recommending this book to friends, colleagues and patients far and wide.'

Dr Hannah Short, GP and Specialist in Menopause and Premenstrual Disorders

Finding Me in Menopause

Flourishing in perimenopause and
menopause using nutrition and lifestyle

DR NITU BAJEKAL MD FRCOG OBGYN

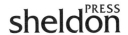
sheldon PRESS

First published by Sheldon Press in 2024
An imprint of John Murray Press

1

This book is for information or educational purposes only and is not intended to act
as a substitute for medical advice or treatment. Any person with a condition requiring
medical attention should consult a qualified medical practitioner or suitable therapist.

A CIP catalogue record for this title is available from the British Library

Trade Paperback ISBN 9781399810227
ebook ISBN 9781399810234

Typeset by KnowledgeWorks Global Ltd.

Printed and bound in Great Britain by Clays Ltd, Elcograf S.p.A.

John Murray Press policy is to use papers that are natural, renewable and recyclable
products and made from wood grown in sustainable forests. The logging and
manufacturing processes are expected to conform to the environmental regulations of
the country of origin.

John Murray Press
Carmelite House
50 Victoria Embankment
London EC4Y 0DZ

Nicholas Brealey Publishing
Hachette Book Group
Market Place, Center 53, State Street
Boston, MA 02109, USA

www.sheldonpress.co.uk

John Murray Press, part of Hodder & Stoughton Limited
An Hachette UK company

To my parents and Rajiv's parents
I know you are looking after us

Contents

Part 3: My menopause

Part 4: Menopause morsels

Note to my readers

I wrote *Finding Me in Menopause* for anyone wanting to learn more about perimenopause and menopause. The book is here to assist you in this important phase in your life, with the help of nutrition, exercise, sleep and other lifestyle factors. It is also for those who wish to learn more about menopause, so they can be of support to their loved ones.

Finding Me in Menopause is not about defining yourself by the menopause or as a menopausal woman. It is about helping you to navigate your menopause journey and make sense of it. Not every sentence, paragraph or chapter will resonate with you and that's because we are all unique, and our experiences of menopause can be vastly different.

This book is for each and every one of you, whatever your age and however you may choose to identify. Perimenopause and menopause are amongst the many phases of life that affect people assigned female at birth (AFAB), including some who identify as non-binary, intersex or transgender for example (**LGBTQIA+**).

When I use the terms 'woman'/'women' in the book, my intention is to include anyone who identifies as a woman or has female reproductive organs, irrespective of gender.

The advice in *Finding Me in Menopause* is not meant to be taken as individualized medical guidance, although it is based on science and the latest research. Using evidence-based, plant-based nutrition and lifestyle approaches, my hope with this book is to guide you to introduce positive changes into your life, however small, with or without medically approved hormone therapy to help you live your life to the fullest.

It is never too early and never too late to learn more about perimenopause and menopause.

Dr Nitu MD FRCOG ObGyn

Please note that the list of references used in this book can be found on the Sheldon Press online library
library.johnmurraylearning.com/ebook/Sheldon-Press/

I am not ready yet: My early menopause (POI)

I looked down in horror, suddenly feeling rather wet. There was blood running down the side of my black trousers, soaking straight through my tampon and super-sized menstrual pad. It was the third day of my period, but I was not prepared for this torrential flooding. I recall being nearly at the end of giving a presentation to ObGyn trainees and consultants on the management of ectopic pregnancy, an area of interest of mine. Horrified, I hurriedly excused myself before dashing off to the bathroom to clean up and stuff toilet paper, a fresh tampon, and a pad into my soaked panties. Waddling back, I took questions on my presentation, without mentioning to anyone what had just happened. Periods and the workplace did not mix together in those days, even in a department that specializes in women's health.

This isn't happening to me

My periods had never really bothered me as an adult, except as a nuisance to be tolerated every month. I had been tracking my cycles, which every person who menstruates should do from the start of their periods right to the very end as periods are an important indicator of one's general and hormonal health.

When I look back, the start of the new millennium was the year my periods started to hop and skip, becoming significantly heavier when they did come, often with clots and flooding. I was just turning 38. Welcome to the noughties.

Within weeks of this incident, the hot flushes and panic attacks took over. I would feel an intense sensation of heat and a creeping wave of fear suddenly wash over me. This happened several times a day and night, without any notice, making me very anxious. I would then go through several weeks feeling normal again, making me doubt myself. Many of you might have experienced this too.

As a junior doctor, well before working hours for trainee doctors were monitored, I worked extremely long hours, doing my best to manage a demanding career and a very young family. My husband and I had no real support network in England, as we were immigrant doctors. I had little time to think about myself, but I do remember thinking, *whatever this is, it can't be happening to me*. I had always placed my health and wellbeing low on my priority list, with no time for self-care, regular meals or downtime. I know this now to be an unhealthy attitude that came at a very real cost to my health and happiness.

Does anyone else think it's hot in here?

After 15 years of strenuous obstetrics and gynaecology training, I was ready to become a consultant, eager to lead a team and put into practice all the knowledge I had gathered over years of hard work. As my periods continued to become erratic, I experienced more of the symptoms associated with **perimenopause** and **menopause** regularly: hot flushes, sleepless nights, anxiety and panic attacks, I had them all. I often had a low mood that was difficult to shake.

I initially put my issues down to the stress of applying for highly competitive consultant jobs, in addition to working long hours and relentless night shifts at the hospital. At the same time, I was experiencing workplace bullying. And so I was not immediately concerned, using all these reasons to justify my erratic periods and other symptoms. Doctors often ignore their own health, to their detriment.

Unknown to me at the time, I was going through a much earlier than expected menopause, known as **premature ovarian insufficiency (POI)**, a condition where periods stop before the age of 40. Older terms for POI, such as 'premature menopause', or 'premature ovarian failure', should be discouraged. The word 'failure' evokes negative feelings and is not in fact accurate; in some cases, a woman with POI may still have some function of her ovaries. The term **early menopause** is used when periods stop between the ages of 40–45. The usual age for menopause is around 51 years, with a range between 45 and 55 years.

My encounter with menopause had started without much notice, and long before I was ready for it. As my mother and older sister had no history of an earlier menopause, there was no reason to think it was on the cards for me. I continued to put my symptoms down to stress, until it was obvious.

Are we ever ready for the perimenopause and menopause? Can we ever be ready for a life-changing event that we have probably heard of but can't imagine will happen to us? In hindsight, my encounter with menopause, at a critical stage on the threshold of my career as an NHS consultant in ObGyn, turned out to be an event that would shape the course of the rest of my life. For this, I am grateful.

Feeling lost

I was used to being in control. This loss of control over my body and not knowing where to turn had a profound effect on me. My periods had stopped so early because of menopause. There appears to be a genetic link in many more cases than we previously believed. Having done some digging in my own family subsequently, this appears to be the case in my situation too, with several cousins in previous generations likely having had POI. *In events beyond my control, my ovaries, dancing to their own beat, had decided it was time to end the party, at just 38 years of age.*

I was now a newly appointed Consultant in Obstetrics and Gynaecology in London, with a bright future ahead, but I can admit now that I was completely lost. As the only woman consultant in my department, I did not feel comfortable discussing my situation with my colleagues, for fear of being judged as weak and ill-equipped in my new role. I wanted to prove myself first at a job that I had worked hard for. I did what many of us do in stressful situations: I buried my head in the sand. Doctors do tend to be not particularly good at seeking help, and I was no exception. I suffered in silence for several years, waiting to share personal information only after I had established myself as a valuable and reliable colleague.

If I had to do it again, I would confide in at least some of my male colleagues, as they turned out to be much more supportive and helpful than I had ever imagined, and became allies. Finding people who can support us in difficult situations can often make the burden easier to carry. *Our friends, family and colleagues cannot help us if they do not know what we are going through.*

Around this time, there was a significant amount of controversy about **menopausal hormone therapy (MHT)**, better known as **hormone replacement therapy (HRT)**, due to possible misinterpretation of the preliminary results reported from the **Women's Health Initiative (WHI)** trials[1,2,3] (see Chapter 3).

Most doctors all over the world were, therefore, hesitant to prescribe HRT medications, including my own family doctor at that time. The truth is that anyone in my situation with POI or early menopause should be investigated in detail by a specialist, and receive the right hormone therapy to prevent long-term issues, except in the few situations where HRT may be contraindicated. This advice has never changed.

We now know, both from newer studies and reanalysis of the WHI trial results, the benefits of HRT outweigh the risks when used for menopausal symptom management, for women, especially in the years around menopause.[4,5] There are some women who have contraindications to HRT. In these individualized situations, it is always best to ask to be referred to a specialist, preferably with a special interest in menopause, so as to receive the best and most up to date advice.

My advice to my younger self, and to anyone in a situation like mine, would be to always seek specialist medical advice – there is help available. Advocating for ourselves is crucial, as being taken seriously can be an uphill battle, especially for women and minority groups. I do wish I had been more vocal about my needs, instead of struggling alone for so long. One of the reasons why I do what I do beyond my clinical work is to hopefully help women avoid being in the situation I had found myself in. Advocating for oneself takes strength. *Women are strong; we just have to remind ourselves of this when society fails to do so.*

What does not kill you can make you stronger

Around a year after my periods had stopped, I turned vegan to support our younger daughter, Naina, who had made up her mind to stop eating all animal products. I saw no excuse to not join her and my older daughter, Rohini, once they explained the facts and their reasoning to me.

As I changed my diet to become completely plant-based, I noted my skin and hair started to glow again, my hot flushes and night sweats got much better. I was feeling so much more energetic than I had in the last couple of years. I explored the culinary world of beans, herbs and spices, feeding myself and my family healthy yet exciting food. I have always loved food, so I cooked and baked with a real passion, as I discovered cuisines around the world rich with authentic plant-based dishes, including my own South Indian culture. My daughters thrived, as did I.

This way of living and eating in alignment with my values sparked my interest in the power of plants, and the significant role lifestyle factors play in women's health. I started keenly observing my patients, becoming very interested in science of nutrition and its effects on the body. *It would take me almost another decade to fully realize that the same healing process that had worked for me could also work for others.*

I had no idea where to access reliable nutrition and lifestyle information that could have helped me when I needed it the most. It meant I had to find out everything for myself. *Surely it should not have to be this way?*

It's never too late

Doctors in the West are not really taught about nutrition, nor that food has anything to do with illness, even though there is so much scientific evidence to support this. Like most doctors, I did not receive any nutrition education during my medical training, either in India or in the UK. *How could this be, knowing what I know now?*

It soon became apparent to me that it is never too late or too early to make lifestyle changes to see benefits for general health, and in all aspects of women's health. As I flourished on a plant-based diet, it made me eager to understand the science behind this way of eating. I loved learning but, as a doctor and surgeon, lifestyle modifications for my patients were something that my attention had never been drawn to, nor had this been part of my curriculum. Western medicine has made huge strides in medical advances, but without addressing our lifestyles, doctors are doing patients a deep disservice.

The missing link

What I discovered, from reading the scientific literature, was that lifestyle is so much more important than I had previously realized. After looking into existing medical trials and studies extensively, I came to understand the critical roles plant-based nutrition and lifestyle interventions play alongside conventional medicine in promoting health.

It seemed so many of the conditions my patients were suffering from would benefit from lifestyle changes. Many of my patients were struggling with hormonal health-related symptoms, from bloating to painful periods to menopausal symptoms, and I started to see real change when they turned their diet and lifestyle around. These changes also helped significantly reduce their risk of other chronic diseases such as heart disease and type 2 diabetes, which often afflicted other members of their family and their communities.

Lifestyle medicine was the missing tool I had been looking for during most of my medical career. Dietary and lifestyle changes can help to prepare all women for many of the symptoms of perimenopause and menopause, and I see this every day in my clinical practice. I now offer all my patients a holistic approach, regardless of whether they need medications or surgery. It's important to remember: *it's not one or the other.*

A light bulb moment

I started questioning the impact I was having, wanting to reach further than my patients. I was keen to share the knowledge I had gained over the years about lifestyle and nutrition.

As it happened, I was invited to speak to a very large group of family physicians on cervical cancer prevention. I arrived early in time to catch the previous lecture on breast cancer prevention. As I listened, there was no mention at any point of the dietary and lifestyle changes one should consider advising all women about with regards to prevention of cancer. There was talk of ultrasound scans, mammograms and fine needle aspiration biopsies – all extremely important for early diagnosis of a cancer that is already present in the body, but not for prevention. Either the speaker felt the doctors already knew about the impact of lifestyle or did not feel it was an important or relevant issue to address. Perhaps they were unaware of the evidence-based lifestyle advice for cancer risk reduction. It was admittedly at a time when cigarette smoking was still permitted in public places, and we as doctors were still ambivalent when it came to advising people on the dangers of smoking, a little like how we still are with alcohol intake (Chapter 15). More on that later.

That evening was enough to make me finally shake off my apprehension as to whether I should make some changes in the way I shared this knowledge. It was not a question of choice anymore. I felt I would be neglecting my medical duty in not educating other healthcare professionals and the public if I did not speak up. I made a commitment to improve women's health through public education and education of clinicians. You will now find me on all social media platforms trying to bust myths and educate people I would normally never have a chance to meet.

Sharing knowledge and raising awareness

I started by approaching several organizations in the medical field as I was already deeply involved in medical education, but no one was interested. The medical establishment was not yet ready to discuss the impact of lifestyle on health. I knew I had to do this, so I set up a voluntary not-for-profit service to empower schoolgirls and women to make informed health choices, while bringing medically proven and reliable lifestyle changes to help better their own lives and, as a consequence, improve the health of their families and the wider community. I wanted these evidence-based lifestyle and nutrition interventions to be available to people of all ages and from all walks of life, not for just the privileged few. Admittedly, this was over a decade ago and I am pleased to say, attitudes have started shifting slowly but surely in the medical community, especially amongst the younger generations.

More exams

I studied lifestyle medicine to further my knowledge and took exams to qualify as a board-certified lifestyle medicine physician, being one of the first to do so in the UK. This expertise, alongside decades of gynaecological experience, has been invaluable in helping me guide my patients and the wider public to make small yet impactful lifestyle shifts.

One size does not fit all

Today, I see amazing improvements in my patients' health and in my family's health when they apply even just a few of the changes that

I discuss in forthcoming chapters. I find meeting my patients where they are at far more sustainable and achievable, rather than simply applying a generic formula.

Had I not been so lost, had I not gone through a much earlier than expected menopause all those years ago, I am not so sure I would have discovered the path to healing myself using nutrition and lifestyle. Finding my purpose in life has been immensely gratifying. I would not change these last couple of decades for anything. Rather than being resigned to commonly held tropes of what menopause and older age hold for you, I hope you, too, will find perimenopause and menopause a time for reflection, for building confidence, for self-care and for defining the new you, as you undertake a journey of self-discovery.

I wish there had been a book that could have helped me during this difficult period in my life. This is why I wrote *Finding Me in Menopause*. I want you to have access to evidence-based information that has the potential to transform your health and that of your loved ones, hopefully well before health issues have taken hold. Just like me, you will find making small changes goes a long way and adds up to a lot very soon.

Today is as good a time as any other to take that step.
Educate, Energize, Empower

For a longer version of my story, visit www.nitubajekal.com

Dr Nitu MD FRCOG ObGyn

A new beginning: Introduction

Your life is not over with the start of menopause, although it may feel like that for some of you when you are in the midst of the changes. In fact, it may just be the start of a new beginning, 'a second spring' for many of you. But you have to prepare for the perimenopause and menopause. This could be your time – whether it was your career, family or life circumstances that meant the years flew by. Perimenopause and menopause can be terribly challenging for many, especially if you are young, but I don't want you to be defined by your menopause, whatever your age.

Unless life decides otherwise, every person with female reproductive organs will experience menopause – that's half the world's population. In fact, there are around 13 million women in the UK alone who are currently peri or **menopausal**, which is roughly one in three British women. In the United States, approximately 1.3 million become menopausal each year. The World Health Organization (WHO) estimates 26 per cent of the global population of women and girls were over 50 years of age in 2021. By 2025, it is estimated that there will be 1.1 billion **post-menopausal** women globally.

Women can expect to live for at least 30 more years after they permanently stop their periods, usually around the age of 51, with life expectancy in women in Hong Kong, Singapore and much of the Western world approaching 83–88 years.

Menopause is the final or last menstrual period a woman will ever have. It is a diagnosis made in retrospect, as it is defined as the absence of periods for more than 12 months. The average age of menopause is around 51 years all over the world, with a range between 45–55 years, with racial variations that I discuss in relevant chapters. Menopause occurs when the number of eggs in the ovaries are depleted enough for menstrual cycles to stop completely.

Perimenopause or menopause in transition is the lead up to menopause. Perimenopause typically lasts for four years, but this can vary between two to eight years.[1] It is associated with hormonal fluctuations, as the ovarian follicles housing the eggs and the production factory of our sex hormones, such as oestrogen, start to decline sharply. Symptoms of perimenopause include hot flushes, reduced sex drive, unwanted weight gain, mood changes that come and go, as do erratic periods which start to lose their usual pattern. For some women, perimenopause may start as early as in their 30s, a time when many women are still thinking of starting or adding to their family.

Menopausal or **post-menopausal** are terms used for the time frame after the 12 months of a woman completely stopping her menstrual cycles. She will remain in this menopausal or post-menopausal phase for the rest of her life. Women often say to me they thought they were done with the menopause. What they really mean is that they are no longer experiencing the acute symptoms, usually hot flushes and night sweats. There are long-term effects of the menopause that we all need to be aware of. I discuss what to expect and how to prepare for these changes throughout *Finding Me in Menopause.*

Part 1 of this book, 'Menopause 101', will help you understand how your **hormones** work and changes the menstrual cycle goes through as you approach menopause. I explain how you can prepare for a doctor's appointment so you can get the most out of it. This setting of the scene is important to help you better understand perimenopause and menopause within the context of the rest of your life.

Menopause can feel like a bolt from the blue

Symptoms of perimenopause and menopause may start long before periods finally stop, impacting both mental and physical health. Few women are told about this, which means they miss out on guidance that could make their lives so much easier. For some women, periods may stop well before they are expected to, as for those with POI (premature ovarian insufficiency) or **early menopause** (Chapter 1).

Eight out of ten women experience several unpleasant symptoms during the menopause, the most well known of which are hot flushes and night sweats, but only three in ten women seek help for them. A great deal can be done through education to empower women well before they approach the menopause.

Menopause is a phase in our lives, where we will hopefully spend several productive decades. This phase is certainly not the beginning of the end, unlike popular misconceptions. Unfortunately, society has made this stage of our lives something to be feared and dreaded. This does not need to be the case. There is help available and women across all socio-economic and educational strata should have easy access to reliable and easily digestible information.

I discuss the benefits and risks of hormone replacement therapy (HRT). There is still a lot of hesitancy among many health professionals and the public when it comes to prescribing or taking HRT, exposing women to misinformation when they would specifically benefit from regulated treatment.

This reluctance to take hormones is largely due to misinterpretation of past studies which suggested a disproportionately higher chance of breast cancer and blood clots than is true for a woman taking HRT, resulting in only one out of ten women who would benefit from HRT actually taking it.

Also in Part 1, I discuss how menopause affects women in the workplace, unwanted weight gain and touch on issues of fertility, contraception and sexually transmitted infections in perimenopause and menopause.

The menopause experience can be different and often negative for people of colour, those who have learning or physical disabilities, LGBTQIA+ people, and those less privileged. I highlight some of the specific hurdles faced by people on the fringes of society.

Whether it is because of lack of access to healthcare, housing or culturally appropriate food, or the many other inequalities present in society, it is impossible to ignore the social determinants of health which impact people, especially women and those from underserved and marginalized communities. We know that health is a privilege in our current world, one which is not available to everyone.

There are other issues in this phase of life. One in three women in the UK are likely to experience a hip fracture and this kind of trauma is very hard to recover from at a more advanced age. Caring about our bones and preventing muscle loss through a number of strategies can stand us in good stead as we get older. I enlisted the help of my husband, Dr Rajiv Bajekal, to write an important chapter on bone health, osteoporosis and muscle wasting (Chapter 5). A senior consultant spinal surgeon, and a lifestyle medicine physician with a wealth of experience,

I could not think of anyone more qualified than Rajiv to write about this crucial aspect of menopause.

It's good we are talking about menopause

There has recently been an interest in menopause in the media and more specifically in menopausal hormone therapy (HRT or hormone replacement therapy), which is encouraging. I am so pleased this dialogue has started. However, reliable evidence-based information that can help us manage our menopause by making simple lifestyle changes is not talked about enough, and often not by qualified health professionals. When there is a lack of communication of reliable health information, confusion reigns.

Lifestyle does matter

When it comes to health, the answer lies more often in our lifestyles rather than just in our genes or in popping a pill. The effects of the food we eat on our physical and mental health is greatly underestimated. As many as one in four deaths is attributed to a poor diet high in sodium, low in wholegrains and fruits, as per the large Global Burden of Disease Study published in *The Lancet* in 2019, that looked at the health of people living in 175 countries.[2] The way we sleep, move, stress, misuse drugs (including tobacco and alcohol) and the relationships we have with our community and environment have far greater impact than many of us, including those of us in the medical profession, would like to believe.

There are robust lifestyle interventions, supported by science and research. However, too many people are coming to harm from not being made aware of the proven simple lifestyle modifications that could help prevent, treat, and manage their chronic diseases. Instead, patients are usually presented with only one standard, pharmacologically driven medical option, because that is the only tool most doctors are equipped with.

Not everyone can take hormone replacement therapy (HRT), not everyone can access HRT, and, more importantly, not everyone wants to. Nutrition and lifestyle advice should be easily available and consistent, with women encouraged to apply it to the best of their ability, whether they choose to take HRT or not.

Part 2 of this book, 'Age-proof your menopause', will give you the exact tools you need to protect the years we live after we stop our periods, without resorting to expensive or unproven methods. There are six pillars of **lifestyle medicine** that are the foundation of all health. I discuss in detail the effects of each of these pillars of health which include nutrition, sleep, stress and physical activity on the way women experience menopause. I explain the science behind the benefits of plant-based nutrition to optimize your health as you approach menopause and beyond. There is a section dedicated to the many benefits of soya for women in reducing hot flushes, breast cancer risk, weight loss and heart health while putting to bed the confusion and myths around the soya bean.

I will have the input of my daughter Rohini Bajekal, an expert nutritionist, board-certified lifestyle medicine professional and author. She answers commonly asked questions regarding the importance of protein in menopause and how to ensure adequate amounts through healthful sources along with other **micronutrients** in the section 'Stronger with age'.

I will also be exploring the place of salt, sugar and oil in our daily diet as well as supplements, as this is an area of great confusion. I discuss the important link between human health and planetary health in light of the climate crisis.

Menopause is big business

About a quarter of the world's female population is set to be experiencing menopause by 2030. At the same time, the global market for menopausal products is growing rapidly, at a rate of more than 5 per cent, rising from its 2021 level of about $15 billion to reach $24.4 billion by 2030.[3]

Menopause is big business for industry. It is important to help people access accurate up to date information, so women desperate for help don't end up getting misleading advice, which could hurt both their health and their bank account. Expensive unregulated bioidentical hormones, useless supplements and unproven salivary, blood or urine assays are just some of the troubling examples promulgated by a multi-billion-dollar supplement industry and so-called 'experts'.

Menopause myth busting

Throughout the years of my clinical practice, and particularly in the last couple of decades, I have listened keenly to the issues my patients commonly face around menopause, and in the years that follow. In Part 3, 'My menopause: Answering your questions', I will be addressing some of these concerns and busting common myths that I hope will be of help to you.

Part 4, 'Menopause morsels', delves into the practical aspects for achieving a sustainable and joyful way of living, with some delicious recipes and top health tips, including recipe contributions by The Happy Pear, with whom I have set up **The Happy Menopause Course**,[4] and Dr Rajiv and Rohini to get you started on adopting the changes we talk about throughout the book.

Feed yourself words of love

Historically, often because of societal stigma, unreliable health advice and pervasive myths, there has been a tendency for women to be blamed or to blame themselves when it comes to health conditions and even natural processes such as menopause.

This persists to this day. Every day I see women, patients, friends and family blaming themselves because of their body weight or their medical condition. I have been no different. It has taken years of work on myself to start accepting my life choices and loving myself for who I am. Speak to yourself as you would to a dear friend or family member. Feed yourself words of love because you deserve it.

Wherever you are in your life right now, I hope to energize you with knowledge around perimenopause and menopause as well as to offer practical advice. My intention always is to share guidance and not to shame you or anyone else about your body, your choices, or your lifestyle.

Life after your periods stop can be productive, fulfilling, energetic and fun. Don't let anyone tell you otherwise. I hope you find the 'menopause mantras' as well as key takeaways throughout *Finding Me in Menopause* helpful.

My sincere wish is that *Finding Me in Menopause* will be a book that you will not only enjoy but hugely benefit from. It can be a resource that you will keep dipping into and will also share with your loved ones. I want this book to be essential reading for you and women of all ages and all stages in their lives, not just those approaching menopause. This is also for anyone who wishes to know how to apply lifestyle interventions and use plant-based nutrition for optimal general and hormonal health, while learning when to seek medical advice.

My aim is to present all the available options when it comes to managing menopause, so you can make an informed decision. In this book, you will learn that lifestyle medicine and conventional Western medicine complement each other.

Nobody knows your body better than you. Nobody loves your body more than you. Whatever your age, get to know your body better. Use reliable health resources to educate and empower yourself. Now is as good a time as any other to start to look after your body as best you can, with the best available scientific evidence. You have this one body so nurture it and nourish it, so it serves you as best it can.

Finally, as a practising senior Consultant Obstetrician and Gynaecologist, with nearly 40 years of clinical experience, having looked after thousands of patients and as a Board-Certified Lifestyle Medicine Physician, I understand the importance of treating women holistically. I would like you to receive the same level of information from myself as my patients, so you can confidently approach your doctor to get the best possible advice for you.

I chose the title *Finding Me in Menopause* for this book as I feel it was through my personal experience with menopause that I truly discovered myself and my purpose in life. I hope it resonates with you too.

With love and sincerity,

Dr Nitu Bajekal MD ObGyn FRCOG Dip IBLM
Consultant Obstetrician and Gynaecologist
Lifestyle Medicine Physician

PART ONE

MENOPAUSE 101 – KNOWLEDGE IS POWER

Perimenopause and menopause may bring a mix of emotions, depending on your own life circumstances. You may feel grief for the loss of fertility, or feel less feminine, especially when you compare yourself to other younger women or look back to your younger self with a sense of loss.

Equally, you may feel relieved that the periods which dragged you down for years have now finally stopped, and an exciting new chapter in your life is about to begin. Any of these, or other, emotions are perfectly normal to experience. In fact, like me you may experience a whole range of emotions over time.

Menopause can be liberating for many women. It is a time when women might be more financially secure, more confident and have no fear of getting pregnant. The ability to say 'no' and not to be taken for granted can be powerful.

My advice as a woman's health specialist with nearly 40 years' experience is for you to empower and educate yourself about your body and the changes it goes through in the course of a lifetime.

This part of the book gives you the basics to help you understand your body, your hormones, defining perimenopause and menopause, how to prepare for a medical appointment and the questions to ask your doctor. I discuss current evidence on hormone replacement therapy (HRT) and its safety. I also highlight two areas that women are most concerned about: weight gain and bone health. In addition to this, I address menopause and the workplace, the menopause experience for people from minority communities, fertility, contraception and sexually transmitted infections (STIs) for women around menopause.

Knowledge is truly power

It can all seem rather overwhelming at first, especially if you have information coming at you from all directions. Misinformation also causes confusion and unnecessary fear. Please don't give up because you will learn in this book how to use evidence-based medical and lifestyle resources. You will have the confidence to engage with your own doctor to confirm that what you understand about menopause is correct and get the appropriate treatment. You will be able to make an informed decision about your health, rather than being put off from seeking helpful medical and health advice because of hearsay and myths. My wish is to educate you using simple language rather than unnecessary medical jargon as this can be rather off-putting.

The way that sensitive and complex issues are communicated matters when health professionals speak to you. Insist that complex medical words and topics are broken down in simple language that you can understand. After all, it is your body that is being discussed and you need to be at the centre of that conversation. Ask your doctor for reliable resources, so you can do some reading or listening to audio sources in your own time. Don't be afraid to correct people gently, including loved ones, if inappropriate terminology or insensitive language are used. Finally, advocate for yourself in all situations.

1

Body works: Changes in perimenopause and menopause

It is important to remember perimenopause and menopause are natural phases in the course of one's life for most women and for those assigned female at birth (AFAB). This, however, is not the case for a significant number of women for whom menopause may occur much earlier than expected for a variety of reasons, impacting health negatively.

It is equally important to be aware that while many perimenopausal and menopausal symptoms may be considered to be a normal part of this phase in life and of ageing, they should not be accepted as such. Certainly not without having access to reliable medical and lifestyle advice, so you can make an informed choice to optimize your menopausal health.

Given that women can now expect to live into their 80s in many parts of the world, thanks to clean water, vaccinations and modern innovations, it has never been more important to prepare for this important phase of life, hopefully spanning decades after your periods stop. I have written *Finding Me in Menopause* specifically to help you on your journey.

This particular chapter may feel a bit medical, but do persevere as it will help you understand menopause better.

Let's start at the very beginning: understanding your hormones

If we are able to understand our body better, it can make us more attuned to the changes it goes through in life. Not knowing the different parts of the reproductive system or how hormones work may cause women to be unnecessarily alarmed in certain normal situations, or equally become complacent when medical help is in fact needed.

A recent survey of 2000 women revealed one in ten women were unable to correctly identify a diagram of the female reproductive system. A quarter of the women surveyed misidentified the vagina and nearly one in two women were unable to properly recognize the neck of the womb (cervix).[1]

You are more likely to receive the correct diagnosis and treatment when you can explain your symptoms clearly when you see a health professional. For example, if you do not know the difference between the **vulva** and the **vagina**, you may be wrongly treated for a vaginal infection, when in reality you may have a vulval skin condition such as eczema or lichen sclerosus. Both these conditions can present with itching, but the treatment is completely different (see Part 3).

The vulva and vagina are often used interchangeably, but are very different parts of your body. The vulva is the external part of the female genitalia on the outside of the body, from the top of the mound or the mons pubis down to the top of the anal opening, and includes the outer and inner lips called the labia majora and minora respectively, the clitoris (the female counterpart of the penis), the vaginal opening or introitus and the perineum. The vagina, on the other hand, is the muscular tube that connects the **uterus** and **cervix** (womb and neck of the womb) to the vulva.

Try to take the time to familiarize yourself, with the help of simple pictures from textbooks or online, of the internal and external female reproductive organs as well as the menstrual cycle to better understand your body. This is so you can recognize when something is wrong and also will help you speak up for yourself with more confidence.

Hormones

You may see the words 'hormones', 'hormonal balance' and 'hormonal imbalance' used frequently in social media and magazines. You may even be confused, as many of these terms are used inappropriately.

Hormones are chemical messengers. The glands and organs in your body that produce hormones are collectively known as the **endocrine system**. These chemical messengers or hormones are released directly into the bloodstream, often travelling to distant tissues and organs to control many important functions in the body, including growth and reproduction.

For example, the tiny pea-sized pituitary gland in the base of the brain releases hormones to control the function of your ovaries located deep in the pelvis. The thyroid is a butterfly-shaped gland located in the front of your neck producing thyroid hormones. The pancreas is a tail-shaped gland situated behind the stomach, producing insulin and glucagon to regulate your blood sugar levels. The two little adrenal glands are triangular in shape and sit one each on top of each kidney, producing important hormones such as cortisol, adrenaline, small amounts of sex hormones, amongst others, regulating our blood pressure, stress response, immune system and other essential bodily functions.

Examples of endocrine or hormone disorders are **diabetes, polycystic ovary syndrome (PCOS)** and those involving the thyroid or adrenal glands (hypothyroidism, Cushing's disease).

The function of ovaries

The main function of our ovaries is the production of hormones and eggs. Women are usually born with two ovaries, the powerhouse of our reproductive or sex hormones (**oestrogen, progesterone** and **testosterone**), although it is possible to lead a normal healthy life even if there is only one functioning **ovary**.

The ovaries, oval in shape, usually the size of a large grape, are tucked low down in the pelvis, close to the delicate flower-like opening of the fallopian tubes, which are attached to the uterus which leads down to the cervix. The egg released by an ovary travels down the fallopian tube each month in the hope of meeting a sperm on its way.

All women are born with a huge number of eggs contained within the ovaries, with numbers anywhere between one to two million. In fact, a woman has the greatest number of eggs when she is a foetus in the uterus. Over time, from the start of puberty and the onset of **menstruation** every month, thousands of these eggs are lost through a process of natural loss or attrition. This decline in egg numbers and egg quality accelerates after the age of 37, all the way through to menopause.

Only about 400–500 eggs will ever be used in a lifetime, with one egg reaching maturity and getting released each month (**ovulation**). There is no way to increase or reduce this natural loss of eggs, unlike sperm in males which is produced every day, with a new sperm cycle from start to finish taking on average 72 days.

Neither taking hormonal birth control (the Pill for example) nor having fertility treatment such as IVF (in vitro fertilization) has any negative impact on the number of eggs in your ovaries or on the timing of menopause.

Testosterone is not just a male hormone

The three main reproductive or sex hormones produced by the ovaries in women are oestrogen, progesterone and testosterone. Their production shares a common pathway involving **cholesterol** produced in the liver, which acts as the building block for these hormones. We do not need extra cholesterol from our food.

There are many functions for these hormones in our body. For example, oestrogen is needed for breast and reproductive organ (uterus, vagina) development in puberty, for regulating the menstrual cycle and for bone, heart and brain health. Progesterone is necessary to prepare the uterus for menstruation and to support pregnancy. Testosterone is needed to maintain normal metabolic function, muscle and bone strength, urogenital health, mood and memory.

Without testosterone, there can be no oestrogen

The levels of these three hormones fluctuate throughout the menstrual cycle and are produced by both men and women in differing amounts at different stages of their lives. A little known fact is that women of reproductive age produce four times more testosterone than oestrogen. Testosterone is in fact the precursor to the production of oestrogen.

We can measure the levels of various hormones in our body by doing various blood, urine and saliva tests at different times of the menstrual cycle. In perimenopause particularly, these tests are not reliable reflections of the true state, as hormones may fluctuate minute to minute, day to day.

The different types of oestrogen

Oestradiol (E2) is the main form of oestrogen in your body during your reproductive years. It is also the most potent oestrogen and is used in modern HRT preparations. After menopause, however, the main form of oestrogen is oestrone (E1), which is much weaker compared to oestradiol, produced mainly by our fat cells and adrenal glands. In pregnancy, oestriol (E3) is the dominant form of oestrogen, synthesized in large amounts by the placenta.

Hormone producers and regulators

Our sex hormones are mostly housed in oocytes or tiny fluid filled follicles containing the eggs within the ovaries. Very small amounts of these hormones are also produced in our adrenal glands, skin, liver, brain and fat cells for example, becoming the main source in menopause, as the ovaries start to shut down. Progesterone is also produced in large amounts by the placenta in pregnancy.

The hormones, **follicle-stimulating hormone** (FSH) and **luteinizing hormone** (LH) produced by the anterior part of the tiny pituitary gland in the brain, in turn control ovarian hormone production and regulate the menstrual cycle. FSH has the job of stimulating ovarian egg follicle development and causing the levels of oestrogen to rise. LH helps in maturing the egg and provides the hormonal trigger needed to release the egg from the ovary to cause ovulation.

The master controller

FSH and LH are in turn controlled by gonadotropin-releasing hormones (**GnRH**), which are hormones released by the hypothalamus, a tiny cone-shaped part of the brain that connects the nervous system to the **endocrine system**. It is like a master switch, allowing hormones to be turned on and off by sending complex messages to and from the brain and pelvis for example. This is why sleep and stress can affect periods and menopause.

The menstrual cycle

The average **menstrual cycle** comes every 25–35 days and is divided into two halves, the follicular phase followed by the luteal phase. In the follicular phase, an egg is selected to grow from the many immature follicles in the ovary in response to the rising levels of oestrogen. The egg is released from the ovary, known as ovulation, in response to a trigger of rising LH. The luteal phase lasts approximately two weeks, as the progesterone levels now rise to help the lining of the womb (**endometrium**) prepare for the implantation of a fertilized egg; in other words, to carry a pregnancy.

If pregnancy does not occur, the microscopic egg is reabsorbed into the body. The levels of oestrogen and progesterone start to fall. This results in blood and tissue from the endometrial lining of the womb to be shed through the vagina, in what we call a period.

Periods

'**Menarche**' is the medical word in Latin used to describe the first ever menstrual cycle or **period**, usually between the ages of 10 and 16. The master switch, the hypothalamus, plays a key role in waking up the reproductive system at this stage in life.

Signs of puberty, such as underarm and pubic hair and breast development, are noticeable a couple of years before periods start. Early or delayed puberty/menarche before age 8 or after age 15 needs medical input sooner rather than later, as there can be health implications.

Bleeding during a period can last between 1–7 days, but should not be longer or painful or heavy enough at any point to interrupt daily activities (see Part 3). If this is a recurring feature, it is best to see a doctor.

Track your periods

Every woman should have her own regular period pattern, unless she is on hormonal contraception when it is absolutely fine not to have a monthly withdrawal bleed.

Every day, I see girls and women from all backgrounds, who struggle to remember their menstrual cycle pattern or the first day of their last menstrual period. This is not highlighted enough in school and college, so women often don't realize the importance of tracking their periods. You too should track your periods from the time you start your periods until you completely stop, either on your smartphone or, if you are worried about digital privacy issues, in an old-fashioned diary. Periods can give us a surprising amount of information about our hormonal and general wellbeing.

Women today can expect to have between 350–500 cycles in their lifetime, depending on number of pregnancies, length of time of breast/chest feeding, hormonal contraception, as well as the age of menarche and menopause.

If you are on hormonal birth control methods, where there is no medical need for a regular withdrawal bleed, I would advise you to be still aware that irregular bleeding or spotting or bleeding after vaginal intercourse should never be ignored in any situation, as most of the conditions causing these symptoms, such as uterine and cervical polyps, infections, precancer and even cancer, can be treated, if caught early.

If your periods are irregular or go missing for more than three months, it is important to seek medical advice, to rule out underlying conditions such as PCOS, thyroid disease, high prolactin hormone levels, eating disorders and **hypothalamic amenorrhoea**. Missed or delayed periods occur naturally for a short while around puberty, in pregnancy and when approaching menopause.

The change in hormones around menopause

In the later reproductive years, FSH levels start to slowly rise, while oestradiol levels remain the same and other hormones such as inhibin (not typically measured) start to decline. The follicular phase starts to shorten (from 14 days to 10 days for example), while luteal phase progesterone levels start to decrease. Even though menstrual cycles may remain ovulatory, fertility potential begins to decline. Typically, a woman is in her 40s when she notices her cycles starting to shorten, although this can vary significantly in individuals.

As the number of ovarian follicles and eggs continue to drop right down as one transitions to menopause (perimenopause), so does the production of oestrogen hormone as well as progesterone and testosterone. These low oestrogen levels in turn trigger a response in our brain, sending messages to the pituitary gland to increase the FSH levels to try to push the ovaries to produce more of the hormones the body needs.

These hormonal changes in oestrogen and FSH are thought to be the driving factors behind the symptoms of perimenopause and menopause.

Empower yourself: Defining and diagnosing menopause

Perimenopause

Menopause transition or perimenopause is the time when a woman transitions to menopause, often marked by hormonal fluctuations. It is that period of time when one moves from having monthly menstrual cycles to a time when periods completely stop. The average age of perimenopause is 47 years and it usually lasts four years, with a range of two to eight years.[2]

The age at which perimenopause starts for a woman depends on when she is destined to stop her periods. If a woman is destined to stop her periods at age 45, perimenopause may start for some women as early as their 30s. Lifestyle, race and environmental factors, such as smoking, body weight or even being Black or Hispanic, also influence the duration and intensity of perimenopausal and menopausal symptoms.

As women head into perimenopause, they may notice initially either shorter intervals, with periods coming more frequently than their previous pattern, or the interval may start to increase to 40 to 50 days. With time, the menstrual cycles progressively become more anovulatory (no egg is released), so women may start to skip periods altogether, sometimes going for months before another period shows up.

Some women will experience heavy or prolonged bleeding at this stage, especially if they have conditions such as uterine **fibroids** or **adenomyosis** or are medically obese. My advice is to always seek medical input in any of these situations, even if it is for reassurance, rather than think heavy prolonged periods are normal and to be expected around menopause.

The menopause: no more periods

Menopause is the *final menstrual period* a woman will ever experience, a time when the eggs in the ovaries drop to such a critical level that menstrual cycles permanently stop. This final stopping of periods also marks the end of the natural reproductive phase in a woman's life.

The average age globally for natural menopause is 51.4 years, with a range between 45 and 55 years of age. It is uncommon for women to have periods after the age of 55 years, with the figure around 5 per cent for women to be still menstruating in their mid-50s.[2,3]

A woman is said to be **menopausal** or **post-menopausal** when she has not had any periods or bleeding for one full year, or 12 months. A woman remains in this post-menopausal phase until the end of her life. Menopause is a diagnosis made in retrospect, meaning on looking back at the previous 12 months.

The first two to six years after the final menstrual period or menopause is referred to as **early post-menopause** and **late post-menopause** thereafter, as per the most widely used and detailed staging system for perimenopause and menopause, known as the STRAW system (Stages of Reproductive Ageing Workshop).[4] It is helpful to be aware of this fact, as some of the symptoms experienced in late post-menopause (usually after six years) are different from those experienced in the first few years of stopping periods.

Factors affecting natural age at menopause

There appear to be racial variations, with South Asian women experiencing natural menopause earlier than the 51 years, even as early as 47 years. Black women tend to have an earlier, more intense and longer menopause while Japanese (East Asian) women become menopausal at a later age compared to their white counterparts[5] (see Chapter 7).

Genetic variations in the oestrogen receptor gene, family history of one's mother's age at menopause and one's own reproductive history are other factors that may also determine age at menopause.[6]

Smoking, including passive smoking, can bring forward menopause by two years.[7] Type 1 diabetes and certain other uncommon conditions (such as galactosemia) may be associated with an earlier than expected menopause. PCOS may delay menopause by about two years.

Night shift work may also have an effect on the age of natural menopause. In a study of over 80,000 women followed for 22 years, those who worked rotating night shifts more than 20 months in the previous two years had an increased risk of earlier menopause compared with women with no night shift work. It is not clear if this effect is related to circadian disruption or to the fatigue and stress associated with demanding night shift work.[8]

Medical and surgical menopause

Menopause is not always natural nor is it always gradual. In fact, it can often be sudden and may come as a shock, even if one is prepared and has been counselled adequately. The perimenopause is cut short, and one is thrown into menopause without much notice to the body.

Surgical menopause is when a woman has surgery to remove both the ovaries whilst they are still functioning properly. This could be for a number

11

of medical reasons, including surgery for certain gynaecological cancers as well as ovarian tumours (benign or cancerous), severe endometriosis, gender reassignment surgery or PMDD (premenstrual dysphoric disorder, a debilitating form of **premenstrual syndrome** or **PMS**).

When medications stop the functioning of the ovaries as a result of chemotherapy, certain other drugs, or radiotherapy, this is known as **medical menopause** and may result in permanent menopause.

Medications such as GnRH analogues (for example, Zoladex and Prostap) induce temporary menopause for a few months and this is different from the more permanent nature of medical menopause. These drugs, when used for a few months as they usually are, are safe, as they mimic the natural hormones released by the hypothalamus. They have been used safely for decades to help with assisted conception, and before or after fibroid or **endometriosis** surgery to help improve outcomes. Menopausal symptoms can be difficult for some women for those months, especially if they have not been counselled properly. Long-term use of these medications in conditions such as severe endometriosis can cause bone loss, so hormones are usually used alongside as add-back therapy to protect the bones.

These GnRH analogue drugs are also used to suppress the ovaries in some women with a diagnosis of oestrogen positive breast cancer, either while waiting for surgery to remove ovaries or on a more permanent basis until age of menopause.

Premature ovarian insufficiency (POI)

Menopause can start under the age of 40 in around 1 in 100 women. This condition is best referred to as **premature ovarian insufficiency (POI)** rather than older terms such as **'premature menopause'** or 'premature ovarian failure'. The latter is both emotive and inaccurate as women may occasionally still ovulate and have periods, with pregnancy rates of around 5 per cent.

Recent reviews of literature show a higher incidence of POI, affecting 3.5–3.7 in 100 women under the age of 40.[9, 10, 11] The age-specific incidence of spontaneous POI is approximately 1 in 250 by age 35 and 1 in 10,000 women under the age of 20.[12]

The condition of POI is characterized by missing periods for more than four months, typically after having had regular periods for a while, symptoms of oestrogen deficiency such as hot flushes, vaginal dryness and night sweats, and FSH levels in the menopausal range before age 40 years on two occasions 4–6 weeks apart.[13]

Causes for spontaneous POI can be idiopathic (where no cause is found) although, increasingly, experts believe there may be a genetic link for many cases of POI. A family member, e.g. sister or mother, with the condition increases one's own risk of POI. Genetic or chromosomal disorders such as Turner syndrome or Fragile X are associated with POI and an earlier age of menopause. Other causes of POI include autoimmune ovarian damage in conditions affecting the thyroid or adrenal glands (examples are thyroiditis or Addison's disease), and infections such as mumps, malaria, cytomegalovirus and tuberculosis.

POI may also be induced because of chemotherapy, surgery or environmental disruptors and smoking.

POI needs to be managed by a specialist team who understand the complexity of the condition, as it is associated with a higher risk of cardiovascular disease, bone loss and cognitive function decline. There is also a significant burden of emotional stress and anxiety from having a much earlier than expected menopause, with implications for fertility and feelings of loss of femininity. Ideally, every woman dealing with POI should be referred to a specialist team and should have access to therapy and counselling.

I highly recommend reading *The Complete Guide to POI and Early Menopause* by Dr Hannah Short and Dr Mandy Leonhardt for an in-depth understanding of these conditions.

Early menopause

This is when periods stop between the ages of 40 and 45 and is said to occur in 5 out of 100 women. Again, this is probably an underestimate, as recent literature suggests a higher incidence of 7.6–12.2 in 100 women.[10,11]

Even these statistics don't consider the many women who have surgical or medical menopause under the age of 45. Studies have shown even a **hysterectomy** (removal of womb) for heavy periods or fibroids, where just the womb is removed and healthy ovaries are conserved in a younger woman, can compromise ovarian blood supply and function, bringing on menopause at an earlier age than the woman was destined for.

Diagnosing perimenopause

If you are above the age of 45 and in good health, a diagnosis of perimenopause can be made with reasonable certainty without the need for blood tests, if you have **vasomotor symptoms** such as hot flushes, night sweats and if they are accompanied by a change in your menstrual cycle pattern. Hormone tests are unreliable in this situation, as they fluctuate too dramatically to be of much help. A blood test done on one day may demonstrate high FSH and low oestradiol levels consistent with menopause, but soon after, FSH and oestradiol may return to the normal pre-menopausal range. Other blood tests such as **AMH** or inhibin are also not helpful outside of research settings in diagnosing perimenopause.

Pregnancy, thyroid issues and ruling out iron-deficiency anaemia by doing simple tests is more important, as well as a pelvic **ultrasound scan** if there are other indications to recommend one such as heavy periods. You also do not routinely need a **pelvic examination** to diagnose perimenopause or menopause unless there are other indications such as possible infections, excess vaginal discharge, irregular or heavy bleeding or pelvic pain.

Diagnosing menopause

If you are seeking medical advice when you have not had a period for over 12 months and you are over the age of 45, a diagnosis of menopause can be made on your symptoms alone (clinical diagnosis) with no need for hormone blood tests. It is important that you take the time to note any other symptoms you may be experiencing and highlight them to the doctor.

Your doctor should ensure that there is no chance of pregnancy and take a detailed medical history. They may then recommend certain tests to rule out other conditions such as thyroid disease, before confirming the diagnosis of menopause.

Diagnosing early menopause

Between 40–45 years, a diagnosis of early menopause is based on some simple, easily available blood tests, which should include hormone levels such as oestrogen, FSH and prolactin levels as well as a full or complete blood count (FBC, CBC) to rule out anaemia and check your thyroid function. It can be helpful to have a thorough pelvic ultrasound scan, ideally a transvaginal scan, as it allows for a closer look at the ovaries and uterus.

It is always important for your doctor to take a thorough medical, surgical, medication and family history and ask details of your clinical symptoms (see Chapter 2).

I would advise referral to an experienced doctor to allow for correct treatment and follow-up for women with a diagnosis of early menopause, along with timely lifestyle advice from an experienced health professional.

Diagnosing premature ovarian insufficiency (POI)

Half the women with a diagnosis of POI have seen three or more clinicians before they receive the right diagnosis. Sadly, one in four women wait for more than five years to be diagnosed, wasting precious time when it comes to optimizing fertility options and preventing heart and bone health issues.

If your periods have stopped for more than four months under the age of 40, after a detailed medical, surgical, medication and family history and examination by your doctor, certain tests should be requested. These include a pregnancy test, a detailed pelvic ultrasound scan, thyroid function, FSH, LH, prolactin levels, with FSH levels of more than 30 IU on two separate occasions 4–6 weeks apart, before a diagnosis of premature ovarian insufficiency (POI) is made conclusively.

With your permission, your family doctor should refer you urgently to a gynaecologist, preferably with an interest in POI, as this needs specialist input and tests. You should have early access to the right medical and fertility advice, reliable evidence-based medical and lifestyle resources as well as patient advocacy groups (see resources).

Referral to a specialist team for consideration of further tests including genetic testing for Fragile X (FMR1 premutation) and Turner syndrome, AMH (anti-Mullerian hormone) blood tests, transvaginal scans to check ovarian egg reserve, thyroid and adrenal antibody tests as well as requesting a **DEXA bone scan** are all part of good medical care for women with POI. Appropriate support, referral to a fertility specialist if indicated, lifestyle and medical advice and choosing the right hormone treatment in the correct doses are critical to prevent long-term complications in those diagnosed with POI.

As POI has serious implications for both short-term and longer-term physical and mental health, a sensitive and empathetic healthcare team is essential. My medical advice is to see your doctor if your periods are missing for more than three months or if they are irregular and outside the 25–35-day interval. This is because there are several other treatable conditions such as PCOS, functional hypothalamic amenorrhoea caused by eating disorders or excessive exercise, and ovarian, adrenal and brain tumours that need to be ruled out or treated early.

Special situations

If you are suffering from menopausal symptoms and you have had a hysterectomy with conservation of ovaries, while you no longer have periods you can still be tested with hormone blood tests. This is because studies have suggested women in this situation develop menopausal symptoms earlier than those who have not had surgery, possibly due to compromise to the ovarian blood supply or by other mechanisms not yet known.

If you are on progesterone-only hormonal contraception such as an implant, the minipill or an **intrauterine system** (for example, the Mirena IUS), then a blood test to check your **follicle-stimulating hormone (FSH)** levels can be helpful to diagnose menopause, especially if you are having symptoms. If the FSH levels are raised, then repeating the test 4–6 weeks apart can help diagnose menopause. If the FSH levels are in the pre-menopausal range, it can be repeated in a year. This is also true if you have no periods after you have had the lining of the womb removed to treat heavy periods, known as an **endometrial ablation**.

If you are on the birth control pill COCP (**combined oestrogen and progesterone pill**), then your doctor will advise you to stop the COCP for 6–8 weeks before checking FSH levels for greater accuracy. You should use barrier contraception during this time to avoid unintended pregnancy. The birth control pill can be continued safely, if desired and after counselling regarding other contraceptive options, until the age of 50 if there are no contraindications and can help with perimenopausal symptoms. For any woman who wishes to continue the Pill after age 50 it is best considered on an individual basis by an experienced doctor.

The expected and the unexpected: symptoms of menopause

You may have heard there are over 34 symptoms of menopause, with hot flushes being both the most well known and the most common of them all. You may wonder whether you will experience all of these 34 symptoms. Most of my patients do not. Many symptoms of perimenopause and menopause may never happen to you or may last only a short while and may also change over time. In fact, there is significant variation amongst women and in different populations as to the number, duration and intensity of menopausal symptoms that one may experience.

The reasons behind menopausal symptoms

Hormonal changes, with a progressive drop in levels of oestrogen hormone produced by the ovaries and rising levels of FSH (follicle-stimulating hormone) produced by the pituitary gland in the brain, seem to be responsible for many of the symptoms experienced by women in perimenopause and menopause.

There is still a lot that is unknown about perimenopause and menopause, and more research is needed in this area to help women manage their symptoms better, with the help of both lifestyle advice and appropriate medications.

After menopause, our body fat and the adrenal glands become the main producers of a much weaker oestrogen (oestrone) rather than the more potent oestradiol produced by the ovaries.

Some of the symptoms experienced in perimenopause can be different from those of menopause. Symptoms of menopause are best grouped into early post-menopause and late post-menopause, although there can be significant overlap.

Symptoms in perimenopause

The average duration of perimenopause is about four years around the age of 47. More than three-quarters of women will notice menopausal symptoms, with one in four women suffering severe symptoms and a third experiencing long-term symptoms.

Period matters

For some of you, symptoms may start just months, and for others, years, before your periods completely stop. You may start to notice shortening of cycles and crowding of periods initially, as hormone patterns start to change, with periods coming more frequently than their usual menstrual pattern. This can lead to feelings of fatigue, with heightening of pre-menstrual symptoms of breast tenderness and mood changes.

Over time, hormonal fluctuations start to get even more pronounced, with longer gaps between periods, often 40–50 days. You may go on to skip periods completely for months at a time, interspersed with normal periods in between, making you wonder what is going on with your body. This is not unusual at all.

If your periods become heavy or prolonged at any point, then iron-deficiency anaemia can become a problem. It is best to seek early medical advice, especially if your symptoms persist for more than three months, if you have heavy or irregular periods or if you have particular concerns about your health.

Fluctuating symptoms

You may notice none, some, or all of these symptoms of hot flushes, night sweats known as vasomotor symptoms of menopause, palpitations (racing heart), disturbed sleep, low mood, headaches, migraines, depression, poor concentration (often described as 'brain fog') and/or lost words or forgetfulness, and a loss of interest in sex or reduced sex drive. New symptoms of breast pain and menstrual migraines may be noticed by some women.

These symptoms may come and go as the reproductive hormones fluctuate wildly at this stage, sometimes on a daily basis.

Early post-menopause symptoms (last 2–6 years after the final menstrual period)

Changes in your hormones can impact both mental and physical health in menopause. All the symptoms experienced in perimenopause, except having periods, can continue into early post-menopause and sometimes even into late post-menopause.

Disturbed sleep

Many women experience problems with sleeping around menopause (Chapter 13). Lack of sleep and fatigue can also make symptoms including irritability, ability to concentrate, stress and anxiety worse. Close to one in two women describe sleep difficulties, especially as they transition into menopause and early post-menopause.

Hot flushes

A **hot flush** (or 'hot flash' as it is known in the USA) is usually described by women as an intense feeling of heat centred on the upper chest and face which spreads all over the body, causing flushing and profuse sweating, and is often followed by chills and shivering, and feelings of anxiety with a racing heart. A typical hot flush may last two to four minutes and can occur several times in a day and night, even every hour, and in some women, just once or twice a day. Night sweats are hot flushes that occur typically at night, and women describe waking up with bed clothes drenched in sweat.

As many as eight out of ten women in the Western world will experience these vasomotor symptoms (hot flushes and night sweats) at some point during perimenopause and early post-menopause. Only two to three women seek medical help, often worried that their symptoms won't be taken seriously or turning to supplements first in the mistaken belief that they are natural, so safer and as effective as regulated HRT.

Women from different countries report different incidences of hot flushes, with 40 per cent of Americans and 52 per cent of Italians reporting moderate to severe hot flushes, compared with only 15 per cent of Japanese women.[14] This may be due to higher fat mass and body weight in the former groups as well as a higher intake of saturated fat (meat, chicken, dairy produce and so on) in the Western hemisphere, with more whole plant foods and **phytoestrogen** intake (beans and soya) in Japanese women and other South Asian women. Smoking and alcohol can also make hot flushes much worse.

Hot flushes usually last for four years or so, but one in ten women may suffer from troublesome hot flushes for as long as 20 years after their final menstrual period.

The more severe these vasomotor symptoms, the more women find all aspects of daily life, including sleep, sexual activity and work, are impacted (see Chapter 6).

The reason for hot flushes

As oestrogen levels drop, the temperature thermo-regulatory centre in the hypothalamus in the brain resets, becoming hypersensitive to very small changes in external and body temperature. There appears to be an increase in the release of norepinephrine and serotonin, which lowers the set point and triggers inappropriate heat loss. That is why certain other drugs, apart from oestrogen therapy, such as **SNRIs** (serotonin-norepinephrine reuptake inhibitors), by rebalancing the serotonin and norepinephrine systems can help reduce hot flushes.

Memory and menopause

Studies have shown women in post-menopause performed significantly worse than pre- and perimenopausal women on delayed verbal memory tasks, and significantly worse than perimenopausal women on phonemic verbal fluency tests (asking women to generate words beginning with a single letter, most commonly F, A and S).[15] Verbal fluency is a cognitive brain function that allows information retrieval from memory. Studies have shown that women in perimenopause can outperform men, so all is not lost. This advantage seems to diminish in later years of menopause.

Oestrogen receptors are widely distributed throughout the brain. Hormones, including oestrogen, can cross the blood-brain barrier by a process called trans-membrane diffusion.

Oestradiol seems to directly correlate to changes in memory performance and function, so low levels of oestrogen are not unsurprisingly related to cognitive changes. Menopause appears to affect how our brain cells are generated and connect with each other and these processes seem to particularly impact regions in the brain that are critical for memory. Menopause also lowers the level of glucose in the brain, the primary fuel used by brain cells, so the brain has to find ways to adapt to the new environment.

Further, women with other medical conditions like diabetes and hypertension are at increased risk for cognitive decline, suggesting similar mechanisms of inflammation and changes in blood supply may be in play both in the brain and the body. Much more research is needed in this area, but it is clear that managing these conditions will protect our brain in menopause. **Alzheimer's disease**, the commonest form of dementia, is sometimes referred to as 'type 3 diabetes'.

Weight gain

Women may start noticing an increase in weight gain, despite no change in diet or exercise. The weight gain appears to be more central, around the middle, with increased internal fat around organs (see Chapter 4). Women may notice a change in their body shape and in their body composition. It can be particularly distressing, as it may be harder to address any unwanted weight gain than it was in the pre-menopausal years.

Depression and other mental health symptoms

Women in perimenopause especially, and in early post-menopause, are at significantly increased risk of depression, compared to women who are pre-menopausal, especially if there is a history of mood disorders (see Chapter 14).[15] Anxiety, irritability, anger and other mood changes are common at this stage.

Joint aches and other symptoms

Joint aches and pain may be reported by one in two women, and more commonly by those who are depressed or carrying **excess weight**. South Asian women seem to experience more of these joint symptoms. Hormonal treatment with oestrogen seems to be of help in these situations. Flexibility exercises such as yoga can also make a difference.

Other symptoms reported by women include ringing in the ears (tinnitus), formication (feeling of ants crawling under the skin), dry hair, loss of scalp hair, increased facial hair, dry skin and brittle nails. The collagen content of skin is reduced in the oestrogen deficient state of menopause, especially noticeable in the later years. Collagen supplements are not particularly helpful (see Chapter 11). Oestrogen therapy may help but again data is limited.

Burning mouth syndrome

This is when women may notice changes in their mouth, lips and tongue, with symptoms such as dryness, burning, tingling, metallic taste, loss of taste, numbness or even pain. These symptoms may be mild or severe, usually short lasting and may come and go, but rarely may persist indefinitely. Menopausal hormonal changes are not the only cause, so your doctor and dentist will need to be involved to rule out allergies, certain deficiencies and to check your thyroid function and medication history.

Late post-menopause symptoms (usually 2–6 years after last menstrual period)

Genitourinary syndrome of menopause (GSM)

Genitourinary symptoms, including vaginal dryness, painful sex, recurrent cystitis and sometimes sexual dysfunction, are most common in the later post-menopausal years.

GSM, formerly referred to as vulvovaginal atrophy, is caused by reduced blood supply to the vulva, vagina and bladder from low levels of oestrogen, causing changes to the labia, clitoris, vagina, urethra and bladder, making the tissues thinner and more easily bruised and sore. You may notice a significant decrease in vaginal lubrication and a feeling of dryness and tightness, with a sensation of paper cuts, especially after vaginal intercourse.

The good news is that these symptoms may respond to a number of methods but especially wonderfully to local oestrogen creams that are safe for almost everybody and can be used indefinitely (see Part 3).

Urinary symptoms such as urinary frequency, urgency, burning, stress and **urge urinary incontinence** as well as recurrent lower urinary tract infections are more common in this stage of menopause. It is important to see a qualified health professional and get treated early and to also follow good bladder hygiene by avoiding soaps and perfumed toiletries in the vulval and vaginal area, drinking plenty of water and seeking medical advice if you notice blood in the urine or burning.

Other long-term effects

There are a number of long-term effects of oestrogen deficiency, including **osteoporosis, cardiovascular disease**, impaired balance and **dementia**. Oestrogen deficiency after menopause may contribute to the development of **osteoarthritis**, but data is limited. These are discussed in some detail throughout the book.

Menopause mantra: *Knowledge is power*

- Understanding the working of our own body and how our hormones work can help us understand the changes in menopause.
- Empower yourself by learning the different definitions of menopause and what to expect.
- Perimenopause and menopause may be natural for many but may occur earlier and be more sudden than expected for others.
- There are over 34 symptoms described and some occur much later in life.
- Symptoms are often varied and are usually linked to oestrogen deficiency and must not be simply accepted if quality of life is affected, as help is available.

2

Being prepared: Questions to ask at your doctor's appointment

For many of us, sitting in front of a doctor can be a daunting experience. I have been on the other side a few times myself, sitting in that chair as a patient. It can be overwhelming, trying to listen intently to everything the doctor is saying, while at the same time worrying whether you have mentioned everything you wanted to. You know you have limited time in your appointment with your doctor, and that in itself can make you appear slow or indecisive when medical or surgical options are rattled off, or a prescription is pushed towards you before you have had time to think things through. Thinking about what you would like out of your consultation beforehand can save valuable time, which can then be used to have a focused discussion about the problem at hand, your menopausal symptoms in this case.

I often suggest to my patients that they write their symptoms down before attending a doctor's appointment, as it can be difficult to remember them all. It is not unusual for your mind to go blank. If you do remember something of importance later, it is good to send that information to your healthcare professional. I also suggest perhaps taking a trusted friend or family member along for support and for a second pair of ears.

A successful consultation

Being ready with the answers to many of the commonly asked questions really helps your treating doctor to give you the right advice and allows them more time to address your current situation. You in turn will feel more satisfied with the consultation.

Your notes should include the following:

- The three top reasons you have made the appointment
- What you would like to get out of the consultation

- Important dates (your first and last menstrual period)
- Details of your periods (flow, duration, frequency, pain, change in pattern)
- Bleeding after sex or in between periods
- Your sexual health history including any infections
- Whether you find sex painful
- Current and past contraception use
- If pregnancy is a possibility
- Cervical smear (Pap smear) screening history
- Results of previous mammograms, bone density if available
- Bring previous medical notes if available
- Have details of your past or present medical or surgical history, bowel and urinary habits
- Family history of POI, early menopause, type 2 diabetes, high blood pressure, heart disease, cancers, and any other relevant information, if known
- Mention any allergies including drug allergies
- Bring a list of current medications and supplements or the actual medication

If you wish to discuss HRT, see Chapter 3 for the questions you may wish to ask your doctor.

If you have concerns regarding your mental health, stress issues, sleep pattern, smoking, alcohol, or other substance use, or any other issue, do bring this to the attention of your doctor as it may have an impact on your treatment options. The information you share with your doctor is confidential and they can help you better if they have the whole picture.

Your doctor may carry out a general physical examination. You may also have your **blood pressure** and other vital signs checked, especially if you are thinking of requesting hormone therapy (HRT). If there is any possibility of pregnancy, bring it to your doctor's notice as you will need a pregnancy test and to discuss possible options.

An internal pelvic examination with verbal consent may be helpful in some circumstances, depending on your answers to the above questions, but is not needed to diagnose perimenopause or menopause. An internal examination is only appropriate if you have ever had penetrative vaginal sex. If you wish for support, a literal or metaphorical hand-hold, ask for a chaperone to be present during any examination, even if seeing a female health professional.

Your doctor may then recommend certain tests including blood tests, a pelvic scan, **bone density scans**, smear tests, vaginal swabs, depending on your individual situation. It is worth asking for specific blood tests such as checking your cholesterol (lipid profile) and blood sugar levels (**fasting blood sugar**, HbA1c) as well as your thyroid function as the risk of serious chronic conditions such as type 2 diabetes, **hypertension** and heart disease starts increasing from the age of 40. These are managed much better the earlier they are picked up.

If you are experiencing heavy or painful periods, bleeding after sex, post-menopausal bleeding, have a family history of early menopause, POI, a personal diagnosis of certain gynaecological conditions such as fibroids, PCOS or endometriosis or if you have had a history of blood clots or cancer, bring this to the attention of your doctor. This is because you will likely need a referral to a specialist for more detailed tests and treatment.

Menopause mantra: *Be prepared*

- Make a list of questions that you want your doctor to answer.
- Be ready with answers to commonly asked questions.
- Take a trusted friend or family member to your doctor's appointment, if possible.
- Consider asking for a chaperone, especially for intimate examinations.
- Be confident and ask the doctor to repeat the answer or break it down into simpler language.
- Request trusted resources for further information.

3

Your choice: Hormone replacement therapy (HRT)

'I feel hot in the day and wake up at night drenched in sweat. I feel more tired than ever, and have a permanent "foggy brain". Everyone is talking about HRT and how good they feel on it. I am nervous about putting hormones into my body, as my mother had breast cancer, and about putting on more weight. I have been taking supplements since my periods stopped two years ago, but I haven't noticed much difference. I want to know if HRT could be right for me.'

Janine, a 54-year-old project manager, had come to see me to discuss HRT. Her main symptoms were frequent hot flushes and night sweats (vasomotor symptoms) that disturbed her sleep and left her feeling tired the next day, unable to concentrate at work. Her mood was often low, and she was upset about the weight gain. Her mother was diagnosed with breast cancer at the age of 75 and died at 90 from a hip fracture and dementia.

Your choice

In a UK survey, 95 per cent of women said they would try alternative treatments before HRT, their reasons being that they think these are more natural and have concerns about the cancer risks with HRT.[1]

Only around one in ten UK women who would stand to benefit from HRT are actually taking it. Some women can't take HRT and others do not want to. It is, of course, always your choice, but I want you to base your decision on scientific evidence rather than hearsay or fear.

In this chapter, I will answer some of the common questions about HRT that Janine and my other patients ask me, which you will hopefully find useful. I will also signpost you to reliable **resources** if you wish to learn more.

What is HRT?

Hormone replacement therapy (HRT) is the use of hormones to relieve menopausal symptoms. HRT is the term preferred in the UK for hormone treatment in menopause, while menopausal hormone therapy (MHT) is the newer, more accurate term and more popular in the USA. Both mean exactly the same.

HRT provides low doses of oestrogen and progesterone (occasionally with added testosterone) for relief of some of the common symptoms, especially hot flushes and night sweats, seen with dropping levels of oestrogen in menopause.

Women need both oestrogen and progesterone combined HRT if the uterus (womb) is still present. Progesterone is needed to protect the lining of the uterus from abnormal thickening (**endometrial hyperplasia**) and from **endometrial cancer**, known risks if the oestrogen were to be used alone. Doses of progesterone need to be adjusted appropriately if oestrogen doses are increased to protect the uterus.

Only oestrogen HRT is needed if you have had a hysterectomy (removal of the uterus and cervix). There are special situations that may need combined HRT for a while such as in some women with severe endometriosis or if the cervix has been preserved in a subtotal hysterectomy.

Is HRT safe?

Yes it is, for the vast majority of women in their 40s and 50s who have no medical contraindications. The advantages of HRT outweigh any disadvantages for this group. Experts all over the world, including the British Menopause Society (BMS), NICE UK, RCOG UK and the North American Menopause Society (NAMS) in the USA, have confirmed regulated HRT is both safe and effective for symptomatic women under the age of 60 years, or if they have been in menopause for less than ten years.

What are the benefits of taking HRT?

HRT is the most effective treatment for hot flushes and night sweats (vasomotor symptoms), the most common and bothersome symptoms of menopause. While systemic HRT is effective for genitourinary syndrome of menopause (GSM), **local vaginal oestrogen** treatment works better for vaginal dryness (see Part 3).

We do not have evidence as to whether HRT can protect against cognition decline and dementia, although there is some emerging evidence that it may be protective when started in perimenopause. If you are looking for specific longer-term situations, such as brain, bone, heart health benefits from HRT, my advice is to have individualized discussions with your doctor. Following lifestyle advice to look after your brain, heart and bones is probably more important.

When should I consider taking HRT?

If you are struggling with hot flushes and night sweats, HRT will almost certainly help you, with noticeable improvements in most women within a few weeks of starting the medications. It can take some adjustment of doses and fine tuning in some cases. Improvement in other menopausal symptoms such as disturbed sleep, mood, fatigue, low sex drive, dry hair and skin changes is variable, with some women finding benefit while others not so much.

It is important to remember hormone therapy will not change life circumstances and your stress, anxiety or depression may be due to other factors. You may need to try other treatment options alongside or separately from HRT, based on your individual situation and your doctor's guidance.

I would advise adopting some or all of the lifestyle modifications that I discuss in great detail in Part 2, as this will help improve your health, regardless of whether you are on HRT or not. A healthy lifestyle will stand you in good stead when you do come off HRT eventually.

Am I a good candidate for HRT?

This is where your doctor comes in. They will take a detailed medical history, ask you about your symptoms, check if there are any specific reasons for avoiding HRT, including your personal and family history, assess your cardiovascular and breast cancer risks, and discuss the various treatment options. If there is any doubt, or there are certain medical concerns, you may be referred to a specialist to help address these specific situations.

It is helpful to be prepared for your appointment by going through my checklist in Chapter 2. Remember to take a list of all your current medications and take your supplements with you for your appointment. This is because some of the supplements and medications you may be taking may interfere with HRT.

When is the best time to start HRT?

HRT seems to be most beneficial for women when started around menopause (perimenopause and early post-menopause), when vasomotor symptoms are common. If you are having bothersome perimenopausal symptoms, you do not have to wait for your periods to stop before you are prescribed HRT. Your health professional will be your best guide after a detailed discussion with you.

Do I need any checks before starting HRT?

Yes, your doctor will take a detailed medical history and do a physical check, including your blood pressure and an internal examination if needed, with your consent. You may be advised to have a **cervical smear** (Pap smear) and/or **mammogram** if you are due one. Your doctor may arrange certain baseline tests (blood, urine, pregnancy test, vaginal swabs, pelvic ultrasound scan), depending on your individual situation.

It is a good idea to request tests to check your blood sugar, haemoglobin and lipid levels, so measures can be put in place in time if problems are picked up.

In general, however, if you are over the age of 45 and there is no doubt of the diagnosis and pregnancy is ruled out, no specific tests are usually needed (see Chapter 1).

What are my options for HRT?

HRT is available as tablets, skin patches, gels or pumps and implants. They all are equally effective. Your doctor will guide you regarding the best option for you, factoring your personal preference. You may try one or two options before you find the one that suits you best.

Common types of HRT

Oestrogen

All types of oestrogen preparations are effective in managing menopausal symptoms of hot flushes and night sweats and should be administered continuously without a break.

- Oestrogen patches/gels/pump: transdermal 17-beta oestradiol is body identical and is like the oestrogen made in our body in the reproductive phase. It is associated with a negligible risk of thrombosis, stroke, and raised triglycerides.
- Oestrogen tablets containing 17-beta oestradiol may be prescribed for women if they prefer tablets to other routes, especially if there are no risk factors. Conjugated oestrogens such as Premarin made from horses' urine are rarely used nowadays in the UK.

Progesterone

Progesterone is needed if you still have an intact uterus and comes in the form of a patch, tablet, coil, pessary or implant.

- Progesterone tablet (body identical): oral micronized progesterone is the tablet of choice with the lowest risk profile for the heart and breast. The daily continuous dose is best for women who have stopped their periods and are a couple of years into their menopause. Younger women who are perimenopausal or have become menopausal recently may have unscheduled bleeding on a continuous regime, so do better with cyclic progesterone for 12 days of each month, which usually results in a scheduled bleed. Vaginal progesterone pessaries are an option if women cannot tolerate oral tablets, although they are currently off licence for use in HRT. In time, women should be switched to the continuous regime from the sequential doses for better uterine protection and to avoid the nuisance of a monthly bleed.
- Progesterone patch: this is used as a continuous combined or sequential combination patch with oestrogen and is usually changed twice weekly. Patches can work well for women who do not want the IUS or the oral tablets. Patches are plant-based with no animal products.
- Levonorgestrel intra-uterine system is a progesterone hormone-containing coil that allows the lining of the womb to be protected

and provides contraception, especially for women who have been started on HRT because of symptoms but have not completely stopped menstrual cycles. The IUS is convenient as it can be left in for a few years, as per manufacturer's guidance in HRT use, with women using the oestrogen gel/patch/spray. It is not licensed for HRT use in the USA.

- Tibolone, a synthetic steroid with oestrogenic, androgenic and progestogenic properties, is another option instead of standard HRT, as is Bazedoxifene/conjugated oestrogen which may be an option for women who cannot tolerate **progestogens**.

Note: I discuss the use of testosterone as part of HRT, low-dose vaginal oestrogen for vaginal dryness and GSM, as well as concerns regarding the use of custom-compounded bio-identical hormones in Part 3.

What dosage of HRT should I start with?

It is advisable to start with the lowest dose of HRT possible and titrating up if needed, to increase adherence by reducing side effects.

Younger women in perimenopause and those having a surgical menopause are exceptions, benefiting from higher doses which can then be adjusted, depending on symptom relief.

What are the side effects of HRT?

Side effects of HRT include breast soreness, water retention and vaginal bleeding. Mood changes and bloating are seen more often with the combined preparations. All these symptoms tend to settle within a few weeks. Vaginal bleeding that is heavy or unscheduled, after vaginal intercourse or if it occurs any time after three months of starting HRT should not be ignored.

HRT has been associated with a small increase in breast cancer, especially with longer duration of use, and a slight increase in blood clots in the first year. With modern preparations of HRT, these risks are minimal under the age of 60.

Will I gain weight with HRT?

There's little evidence that HRT makes you put on weight. I discuss weight gain in menopause in detail in Chapter 4.

Are there any contraindications to HRT?

A history of cancer (especially breast or womb) is usually a contraindication for HRT. If hormone therapy is to be used, this would be a specialized decision made by a team of experts.

Similarly, a personal history of thrombosis is considered a contraindication for HRT. With a family history, certain tests may be needed before starting HRT. A history of existing heart disease (ischemic heart disease, peripheral arterial disease) is considered a relative contraindication for the use of HRT. Any hormone treatment in these situations must be individualized with specialist guidance and advice. There are other potential medical contraindications which are also best managed on an individual basis.

What about HRT in POI and early menopause?

In these situations, women should be on the right doses of HRT from the time of diagnosis until at least the average age of menopause (51), with annual reviews. Bone and heart protection are particular concerns in these women, so HRT is recommended unless there are specific medical reasons not to take it. An individualized decision should be taken if using the combined hormonal contraceptive pill instead of HRT for women with POI who wish contraception.

Compliance with HRT

When women do start HRT, compliance may be poor, with more than half stopping within one year of starting.[2] There are a number of reasons for this:

- Failure of the health professional to clearly explain the benefits and risks as well as possible side effects of HRT
- Unwanted side effects such as breast tenderness, bloating or vaginal bleeding that would normally settle in a few weeks to months of persisting with HRT
- Confusion after reading or hearing concerns about safety of HRT
- National shortage of HRT preparations
- Unrealistic expectations of what HRT can do.

HRT hesitancy

Many women remain anxious about taking HRT even today, when they would benefit hugely from taking hormones to get safe and effective relief for their menopausal symptoms in their 40s and 50s. Initial misinterpretation of the results from the large WHI trials has been partly responsible for this. Despite evidence to the contrary after reanalysis of results[3] and newer studies confirming the safety profile of HRT in younger women, public and medical opinion has been slow to change, with negative consequences on women's menopause experience and quality of life.[4]

The WHI HRT trial controversy

HRT started in the 1960s and became very popular in the 1990s. The Women's Health Initiative (WHI) hormone therapy clinical trials recruited around 27,000 women from 40 clinical centres in the USA between 1993 and 1998 to test the effects of post-menopausal HRT on the risks of coronary heart disease primarily, as well as on hip and other fractures, breast cancer and in those women with an intact uterus, uterine cancer.[5] Between 1996 and 2001, in the largest study of its kind, the Million Women Study in the UK invited women aged 50 and over for breast screening and analysed their health data.[6,7]

In July 2002, around the time when I was seeking HRT for my earlier than expected menopause, the preliminary results from the WHI trial and the Million Women Study stated that HRT had more risks than benefits for all women, including the risk of developing breast cancer whilst on HRT. These results received worldwide coverage, creating panic amongst care providers and the public. New guidelines were drawn up and both HRT prescribing and use dropped dramatically. The trials were stopped earlier than planned.

There had been a misinterpretation of initial results when announced in a press release and at a press conference, as well as a failure to highlight that the group with a higher incidence of cardiovascular disease and breast cancer were in fact far older than the population (60s and 70s in the US study) for whom HRT is normally prescribed (40s and 50s).

Breast cancer and HRT

In 2020, the final results of the WHI clinical trials of the women followed from the 1990s to 2017 were published.[8] The study found that women who took oestrogen-only HRT were less likely to be diagnosed with breast cancer or die from breast cancer than women who did not take any form of HRT. There was a small increased risk of breast cancer associated with combined HRT, but no increased risk of death from breast cancer in these women.[8]

About 2 in 100 women using combined HRT will develop breast cancer that they would otherwise have avoided. The risk of breast cancer persists for a while after stopping HRT and the risk is doubled if the duration of the use of HRT is ten years compared to five years.[9, 10, 11] This risk is mostly from the progestogens used in combined HRT to protect the uterus.

To put these risks into context, 8 in 100 breast cancer cases can be attributed to alcohol intake and another 8 in 100 to increased body weight, compared to 2 in 100 from HRT. Another study found that in recent oestrogen-only HRT users, between 3 (in younger women) and 8 (in older women) extra cases per 10,000 women years would be expected, and in oestrogen-progestogen users between 9 and 36 extra cases per 10,000 women years.[12] The risk seems to be mainly for older women and for those using HRT for long durations (ten years or more).

HRT when used for five years in women in their 40s and 50s comes with negligible increased breast cancer risk. Similarly, those with POI (under 40) and early menopause (under 45) are not considered at increased risk. There is some data to suggest that micronized progesterone may not be associated with an increased breast cancer risk.

Can I start HRT if I am over 60?

Starting HRT ten years or more after your periods have stopped or above the age of 60 is generally not advised. That is because of concerns about increased breast cancer risks with increasing age. However, hot flushes are still an issue for one-third of women ten years after the final menstrual period, with 8 in 100 women having hot flushes more than 20 years after menopause.[13, 14] Hormone therapy can still be considered for this age group after a detailed discussion, ideally with a doctor experienced in treating menopause. More studies are needed in women who start HRT after the age of 60, but early reports suggest they are safe.

How often should I see my doctor when I am on HRT?

A yearly check with your doctor is advised after an initial review in three months. An annual review of your health and your medications is important, with laboratory tests and pelvic scans as indicated. You should seek urgent medical advice if you have any unscheduled bleeding, if your medications are not working, your situation changes or if you have concerns. Do ensure you are up to date with your screening, including your cervical smears, mammogram, bowel health check, as appropriate. Try to keep up with lifestyle changes alongside HRT.

How long can I be on HRT and will my symptoms return on stopping?

Women can be reassured that the absolute risk of complications for healthy, young post-menopausal women taking HRT for five years is very low.

While women can take HRT for as long as they find it beneficial, my advice is to review the situation yearly to help the woman decide if she wishes to continue HRT. I have found it is better to wean off gradually over a period of 6–12 months in most situations. However, some women may prefer to stop HRT without weaning. Studies haven't shown benefit one way or the other.

For many women, symptoms do not return after stopping HRT, especially if they have put lifestyle measures in place. If menopausal symptoms return after stopping HRT, non-hormonal measures should be offered first, but if women wish to consider restarting it and, provided they are fully informed of the risks, HRT should not be withheld.

Are there alternatives to HRT?

If you are considering supplements and certain other alternative treatments, do involve your doctor, as there may be drug interactions, and always seek the advice of qualified health professionals.

In general, the evidence is not strong for herbal and botanical medicines for effective relief of menopausal symptoms when compared to HRT (see above). Look for the THR logo standing for traditional herbal medicines that have been approved for their dosage,[15] quality and product information, as most herbal medications are unregulated with unpredictable doses and purity.

Complementary therapies are treatments used alongside conventional medicine. For example, hypnosis for hot flushes, mindfulness-based interventions, yoga, aromatherapy, **acupuncture** and acupressure may be used to provide some relief of menopausal symptoms, either alongside or instead of HRT.

Alternative medicine uses a different approach from conventional medicine. Large trials with robust evidence are lacking to endorse ayurvedic and homeopathic treatments for menopausal symptoms.

Non-hormonal medical treatments

Certain medications such as antidepressants (**SSRIs**, SNRIs) or gabapentin or clonidine may be options for women who cannot take HRT. Fezolinetant, a neurokinin 3 (NK3) antagonist, is a new non-hormonal medication that has been approved by the FDA to be used for treatment of moderate to severe menopause-related hot flushes. It works by restoring the balance between oestrogen and neurokinin B (NKB) by blocking NKB in the temperature control centre of the brain. Additional trials are recommended before they are recommended widely. All these medical treatments must be prescribed by a qualified doctor.

Case outcome: After a thorough consultation and informed discussion, Janine opted for the continuous combined HRT patch alongside lifestyle advice with a nutrition professional, in view of her raised **BMI** in the overweight category. I gave her resources, including fact sheets on my website, to read to inform herself more about menopause and HRT. She was aware of the possible side effects and when I saw her three months later, she was very pleased with her symptom management with both HRT and the lifestyle advice. I discharged her back to her GP to be reviewed on an annual basis unless there were any concerns earlier.

Menopause mantra: *HRT is safe and may be right for me*

- HRT is the same as menopausal hormone therapy (MHT).
- HRT is the use of hormones to relieve menopausal symptoms.
- Oestrogen-progesterone combined HRT is prescribed in women with a uterus.
- Oestrogen-only HRT is used for women who have had a hysterectomy.
- Testosterone may be considered for some women.
- HRT is most effective for managing hot flushes and night sweats.
- HRT is safe for the vast majority of women in their 40s and 50s, with no medical contraindications, when prescribed under 60 or within ten years of menopause.
- The risk of breast cancer is minimal in this group, with two extra cases in 100 from taking HRT compared to eight in 100 from alcohol intake.
- If a woman wishes to continue with HRT beyond five years, it must not be withheld, after thorough counselling.
- Local vaginal oestrogen is safe and effective for vaginal dryness.
- Lifestyle advice must be given alongside HRT.

4

I eat the same, I weigh more: Weight gain in menopause

'Nothing seems to fit anymore.'

'It is as if my body shape has changed in the last few years.'

'I seem to have this permanent muffin top.'

'I can't stand to look at myself in the mirror.'

'If only I could lose another few kilograms, I would be so happy.'

I hear these and many more similar statements from my patients and women I speak to. Weight gain is probably one of the more common symptoms that women say they struggle with in perimenopause and menopause. Unwanted weight gain can be frustrating at any age, and women understandably want answers and quick solutions, the latter not being easy to come by.

> 'You have to be thin, but not too thin. And you can never say you want to be thin. You have to say you want to be healthy, but also you have to be thin.'

These words from the brilliant monologue by America Ferrera, acting as Gloria in the movie *Barbie*, should make us pause for thought and think of the unrealistic and oppressive beauty standards we have as a society.

Societal expectations of being slim as a woman seem to be almost a prerequisite for physical beauty in most parts of the world. It is little wonder that many women are permanently on some diet or other that promises weight loss quickly and easily. Chasing this illusion of a perfect body, surveys have shown over half of women are trying to lose weight, with two-thirds saying they do so most of the time, with a significant impact on their mental health.[1,2,3] Yo-yo dieting leads to further increases in weight over time.

My advice for you is to try to change the narrative and speak to yourself with kindness. While there are many health benefits of losing weight when one is medically obese or overweight, losing weight should never come at the cost of your mental wellbeing.

I hear so many women of all ages speak about themselves in a self-deprecating manner, with disgust and dismay. Perimenopause and menopause are difficult enough at the best of times, so avoid putting undue pressure on yourself to lose weight at any cost. It is perhaps the time to learn to accept yourself and gradually shed that negative body image of yourself.

I am fully aware that 'body positivity' is a term that some people believe is often overused. I, for one, firmly believe that we as a society have to do everything to encourage people to feel good about themselves and the physical body they are born with. If it means embracing the term 'body positivity', then I am all for it. Body neutrality, or the ability to accept and respect your body even if it isn't the way you'd prefer it to be, might be a less daunting goal. The goal of body neutrality is to feel at peace with your body, reminding yourself that self-worth is not centred on your body's appearance.

I hope you find the ways I suggest, and other methods, helpful for you to achieve the same goal of weight loss, but with fewer negative feelings attached to it.

Weight gain with age

Most adults tend to steadily put on weight between the ages of 20 and 65, with women putting on more weight than men over a ten-year period, especially in midlife. Data from the USA shows weight gain is greater in Black women compared to other races, with less weight gain noted in East Asian women.

Genetic factors play a role in weight gain but it is important to remember, diet, lifestyle and environment are more important factors than genetics for most people.[4]

Total weight gain around menopause

Women in their 40s and 50s, as they approach perimenopause and menopause, gain on average 0.7 kg (1.5 pounds), independent of their initial body size or race or ethnicity.

In the USA itself, nearly two-thirds of women aged 40 to 59 years and about three-quarters of women 60 years and older are medically overweight, with close to half being classified as medically obese (BMI greater than or equal to 30 kg/m^2).[2] The statistics in the UK and around the world in high- and mid-income countries are not much different.[5,6]

Under the skin

There also appears to be more of an increase in the fat you cannot see or the internal visceral fat, often associated with health conditions such as **metabolic syndrome** and type 2 diabetes, as well as weight around the middle (central fat distribution).

As part of the large US Study of Women's Health Across the Nation (SWAN) that spanned several years, interesting insights were gained into the changes in body weight and body composition of 550 multi-racial women, initially aged 42–52, as they went through menopause. Around two years prior to the final menstrual period, the rate of fat gain was found to double, and lean mass started to decline, and this continued until two years after the final period (menopause). Women gained an average of 2.9 kg, with a 3.4 kg increase in fat mass and corresponding loss in lean muscle mass, and a 5.7 cm increase in waist circumference in the six years they were followed.[7] The rate of waist circumference increase slowed one year after the final menstrual period, whereas fat mass continued to increase without change. Many women say they put on even more weight than this.[8,9] Weight gain of 3–10 kg is not uncommon around menopause.

Change in body shape

Using BMI (Body Mass Index), a measure that uses your height and weight to work out if your weight is healthy, is not particularly helpful in women in perimenopause and menopause. BMI is not able to especially predict type 2 diabetes or cardiovascular disease, as it's the body composition that also changes in menopause, with an increase in fat deposition and concurrent loss in lean mass, and not just body weight.[7] Women in menopause say their entire body shape has changed compared to their younger years.

Reasons for weight gain in midlife

Apart from getting older, there are several other reasons why women put on more weight in the years around menopause. Some of these are under our control, but many are not.

The increased levels of FSH (follicle-stimulating hormone) seen with menopause may be independently involved in this weight gain and may be in fact an important factor, separate from the dropping oestrogen levels seen around menopause, but more research is needed in this area.[7,10]

Sleep disturbances become common as the reproductive hormones fluctuate in perimenopause and menopause, with hot flushes and night sweats waking women up at night. Even without oestrogen levels dropping to cause sleep issues, anxiety, depression, stress and restless leg syndrome can all keep women awake at night. Sleep deprivation and poor quality sleep both make it easier to put on weight and harder to lose it once it is on.

Because of timing, menopause often coincides with other life changes such as unwell relatives or parents, children moving out and relationship problems, making it harder for women to maintain positive lifestyle behaviours, becoming more sedentary and turning to comfort foods, resulting in further weight gain.

The menopause transition for women often comes at a time in one's life where one may be eating out more often, consuming more calorie-dense foods, higher in salt, sugar and fat, as well as drinking more alcohol. All these add to gradual increases in weight over time and make it harder to shift.

Hormone replacement therapy and weight gain

Contrary to belief, several studies have failed to confirm a link between weight gain and the use of HRT. Oestrogen therapy also does not seem to prevent weight gain in menopause, although it may minimize fat redistribution and maintain more lean mass. It might be because oestrogen replacement does not completely suppress FSH levels, which as explained above may be a contributor to the weight gain seen around menopause.

The best diet

Getting into an energy or calorie deficit is the single most important factor needed for weight loss. Current evidence suggests that no single diet has been found to be better than another for short-term weight loss. Every single diet, although their names and approaches may change with time (Atkins, Paleo, South Beach to name just a few), works on the principle of reducing calories, often focusing on increasing or reducing single macro constituents of diet (protein, fat, carbohydrate) such as an animal-product derived ketogenic or low-carb, low-fat or high-protein diet. These can work in the short term, although the potential risks to our health and long-term effectiveness remain unknown, with initial reports suggesting possible harm.[11,12,13]

Achieving long-term weight loss

There is a lot of societal pressure in high- and middle-income countries for women to have a particular shape of body, usually tall and skinny. This is not a realistic expectation for most women, and is doomed to cause unhappiness, while the diet industry is laughing all the way to the bank. Embracing the changes your body goes through in perimenopause and menopause is important for your mental wellbeing, as there are many aspects of weight gain that are beyond your control.

If you however do wish to aim for long-term sustainable weight management, a Mediterranean-style plant-predominant or plant-exclusive diet will always win hands down. This way of eating that is rich in whole plant foods (Chapter 10) is naturally lower in calorie-dense foods, low in saturated fat and refined carbohydrates but nutrient dense, keeping one satiated. It is also a joyous and abundant way to eat. People always tell me later how mistaken they were in thinking that a plant-based diet was one of restriction and deprivation. Eating should be pleasurable, not associated with guilt.

Wider benefits of using plants for weight loss

A **whole-food, plant-based (WFPB)** diet does not need you to count calories, which is in itself tiring, while helping maintain sustained weight loss, improving not just BMI but also cholesterol and blood sugar levels, reducing your risk of type 2 diabetes, obesity and ischaemic heart disease amongst other chronic diseases.[13,14]

It really is fundamental that you adopt a diet that creates a calorie deficit (negative energy balance) while prioritizing nutrient quality to promote health.[15,16]

Losing weight at a cost to your health is never worth it.

Other considerations

Studies suggest meal timings are also an important factor in weight loss and management, so do consider eating in tune with the circadian rhythm, with larger meals earlier in the day.

There is some evidence of variable quality to suggest alternative approaches such as yoga and acupuncture may also aid in weight loss.

Weight loss medications and surgery

The impact of menopause on gut hormones, such as leptin, ghrelin and adiponectin, that regulate satiety, remains unclear. A wide variety of medications is available to suppress appetite, promote satiety and target **insulin resistance** with resulting weight loss. These drugs are not without side effects, and usually need to be taken long term.

My advice is to always seek help and support from a qualified medical professional before commencing these medications or considering bariatric surgery, all sensible options for the right patient but needing an informed decision. Self-prescribing these medications can be counterproductive and in some cases harmful, so do avoid buying weight loss drugs of questionable quality online. Lifestyle changes should be adopted before or alongside medications for long-term success. Further discussion on this topic is beyond the scope of this book.

Helping yourself

There is no quick fix for weight loss and whatever the advertisements tell you about new fad diets or diet supplements, they do not work in the medium or long term. They may also harm your health. Focus on good health with a nutritious diet and regular exercise, rather than a perfect body weight. Being slim does not always equal healthy and vice versa. It is much more than that.

Find your why

Behavioural changes are important if you want sustained weight loss. Rethinking your relationship with food and changing your mindset are likely more important than any other factor in keeping weight off. Ask yourself why you want to lose weight.

Weight loss goals for the vast majority of people are destined to fail. Instead of setting yourself weight loss targets, my suggestion is to set yourself goals that resonate with you. For example, they may sound like this:

'I want to get stronger.'

'I want to get fitter so I can travel.'

'I want to reduce my risk of chronic illness.'

'I want to be able to play with my grandchildren.'

'I want to have more energy when I go for a walk.'

Consider front-loading your calories with breakfast and lunch being the more calorie-dense meals. Finishing your evening meal by 6–7 pm, in combination with overnight fasting, may help you in maintaining weight loss. Mindful eating, smaller portion sizes and restricting certain snacks will all help.

Avoid crash diets. Instead consider keeping a record of your calories, perhaps using a smartphone app such as Cronometer at no cost, for a week or so and maintain a steady loss by reducing approximately 500 kcals daily from your 1700–2400 daily calorie requirement, depending on your age, weight, physical activity etc. Avoiding any of these will slash your calories by around 500 calories: a shop-bought frappé, a doughnut, a bagel with cream cheese, a meat-based burger, bacon slices or a chunk of dairy cheese. Alcohol can also be a source of empty calories and can add up pretty quickly, with zero health benefits.

Adopting a plant-exclusive or plant-predominant diet will help you do this healthfully and much more easily.

Regular exercise can help maintain weight loss achieved through changes in diet. Strength training is especially helpful in preventing loss of lean muscle mass and for building muscle.

Ensure you find the support you need to help you, by either finding a friend or family member, an online support group, nutritionist or dietitian, even smartphone apps, as positive encouragement will help you achieve your goals.

Lifestyle modifications in managing stress, sleep and avoiding alcohol along with dietary changes and physical movement all have a role to play in helping women maintain a healthy body weight as they approach menopause. I discuss each of these lifestyle factors in detail in Part 2.

Menopause mantra: *I am more than my appearance, weight and shape*

- Weight increases steadily from age 20 to 65.
- Women put on more weight than men, with weight gain of 3–10 kg around menopause.
- Yo-yo dieting leads to further increases in weight over time.
- There are changes in body shape and composition with more fat around the middle.
- There is an increase in internal visceral fat in menopause that increases risk of chronic illness.
- There is significant loss in lean muscle mass with corresponding increase in fat deposition.
- All diets work on the principle of reducing calorie intake, remembering there is no quick fix.
- A diet rich in plants is both calorie light and nutritionally complete and allows for short- and long-term healthy weight loss.
- Use all lifestyle pillars and set health-related goals rather than weight loss goals.
- Be kind to yourself and find a support network.

5

Strong to the core: Preserving muscle and bone health

Dr Rajiv Bajekal, consultant spinal surgeon and back specialist

For close to 40 years of my life as an orthopaedic surgeon, my main role in **osteoporosis** was at the point when I saw a patient who had sustained an osteoporotic fracture of the hip or spine. I would be involved in the surgical treatment of these fractures. After I developed an interest in lifestyle medicine, I realized a lot of what I saw could be prevented by simple lifestyle changes, particularly before these fractures occurred, but also after a fracture occurred, to prevent another one.

Most people are unaware that for both women and men, bones are at their strongest in young adult life. In fact, bone loss starts as early as our mid-30s, accelerating in women as they transition to menopause and post-menopause. This is a result of the hormonal changes that directly affect bone density. Both oestrogen and testosterone are needed for strong bones and these levels fall significantly in the years around menopause and after.

A substantial amount of bone loss of around 3 per cent or so of the total bone mass is lost in the year around menopause. The annual rates of bone mineral density loss appear to be highest during the one year before the final menstrual period and through to two years after (early post-menopause). This can have serious consequences, as bones become fragile and prone to fractures, unless one starts with more bone stock in the 'bank', i.e. more reserve before this period in one's life. However, it is never too late to start taking measures to strengthen your bones.

Bone is living tissue

Osteoporosis is a disease that makes bones weak, with an increased risk of fractures, especially of the spine, wrist and hip, often known as fragility fractures, meaning fractures that occur from standing height or minimal trauma. The bones become thin and brittle, as new bone is not laid down quickly enough to keep up with the old bone that is constantly being broken down and replaced throughout our lives. Bone is not static but is being constantly remodelled, as it is a living tissue.

The risk of osteoporosis is increased in menopause, especially if there is a history of early menopause or a hysterectomy under the age of 45 (particularly if the ovaries were removed), resulting in low levels of oestrogen, which protects bones. Women who have been on long courses of steroids for other medical conditions, or have been bed-bound for prolonged periods due to illness, or have a history of eating disorders such as anorexia nervosa (resulting in severe calorie restriction) or of exercising so much that periods stop (hypothalamic amenorrhoea) are at greater risk of developing osteoporosis or weak bones. Robust studies have confirmed oestrogen as the treatment of choice for preserving bone strength and preventing osteoporosis in menopause, especially those with POI.

Consequences of osteoporosis

Osteoporosis is a painless condition, until a bone is fractured. In fact, even after certain fractures (e.g. of the spine) there may be no pain at all (60 per cent of vertebral fractures can be painless) and therefore the condition may not be recognized until more serious hip fractures occur.

Hip fractures, often after a minor fall, can severely affect physical mobility in many women in late post-menopause. Type 2 diabetes, hypertension and previous stroke further increase risk. Early mobilization with exercises supervised by qualified physiotherapists and early discharge from hospital along with social and medical support at home allow for a quicker return to normal life. HRT reduces the risk of both spine and hip fractures, so should be part of the discussion in those at high risk of osteoporotic fractures.

Strong muscles

Bones are supported by muscles and ligaments, so strong muscles provide good support to our bones. Sarcopenia, or muscle wasting, and osteoporosis often tend to go together, so measures should be taken to improve both muscle and bone strength to reduce the risk of these conditions that significantly compromise quality of life in later years.

Measuring osteoporosis

The most accepted current method is a DEXA scan. While this is not a true bone density measurement, it is simple, involves minimum radiation, is reasonably well standardized and generally readily available and affordable. DEXA scans compare your bone density to that of others in the population.

There are two scores to focus on in the report.

- The T-score compares sex and race-matched individuals to a young individual aged around 30.
- The Z-score matches sex and race-matched individuals of a similar age.

T-scores of −1 to 1 or above are considered to be 'normal'.

T-scores of −1 to −2.5 is osteopenia (weaker than normal but not yet osteoporotic).

Below −2.5 is considered osteoporotic.

Z-scores should generally be −2.5 to +2.5.

Using lifestyle to get strong

Studies have shown it is never too late to start building strong bones and muscles, with even women in their 70s significantly reducing their risk of getting a hip fracture by making changes in their diet and exercise. Those who make the most changes seem to have the greatest benefit.

A team effort

From a practical perspective, it is important to understand that bone is a living 'structural tissue' and responds like other tissues in the body to changes in nutrition. Like your muscles, it responds to mechanical stimuli and becomes stronger with loading. Bone and muscle strength is therefore a team effort between diet and exercise.

A new skeleton

It stands to reason that the more bone we have at a younger age, the better it is for us as we get older. Balance in the bone remodelling process is important, and too much bone loss in the absence of bone formation will cause osteoporosis. Did you know we replace our skeleton every ten years?

Exercises for bone health, muscle strength and cognition

As we discuss in Chapter 19, the chapter on exercise, body weight exercises and resistance training using resistance bands or dumbbells (initially under supervision, if new to these exercises) are very effective at improving bone strength and muscle strength. A minimum of two strength training sessions of 30 minutes each per week is recommended to preserve bone and muscle mass. Walking does not by itself increase bone strength, so consider using a weighted jacket or strap-on wrist or ankle weights to mechanically stimulate our skeleton to form new bone.

Activities such as skipping, jumping jacks, burpees etc. are free to do, with no added costs, and can help strengthen your bones. Running is curiously not as effective as resistance training in improving bone strength and muscle strength. (This may be because runners are generally slimmer and this activity loads bone only in one axis.) Swimming and cycling, while being excellent forms of exercise, are not anti-gravity exercises and so do not help directly in improving bone strength.

It is best to do a variety of exercises as bone is a three-dimensional structure and loading it from different directions improves bone strength. Flexibility, balance and posture exercises such as yoga and tai chi are particularly helpful for women as they grow older, helping to reduce falls.

Muscles also form communication molecules called myokines and these are known to even help cognition and prevent dementia.

Adequate sleep and rest between days of training are also key to the process of building stronger bones and muscles. This is because exercise is in fact a stressor we place on our bodies, although with good consequences.

Recommendations for exercise in osteoporosis

Osteopenia and osteoporosis are lifestyle conditions, and it is best to manage them by making changes in your lifestyle rather than by medication alone. If you have been diagnosed with severe osteoporosis, I would recommend an exercise programme under the supervision of a qualified health professional and gradually stepping it up.

Dietary factors for strong bones

Bone formation requires several **macronutrients** and micronutrients and not just calcium and vitamin D, as you may have been led to believe. While calcium is clearly an important micronutrient, bone is not chalk and it is too simplistic to elevate one mineral to the high altar that calcium has been raised to.

Macronutrients for bone health

Protein

Bone formation depends on an adequate supply of amino acids which are the building blocks of proteins that go into bone formation. Proteins are essential to bone formation, with most healthy adults needing around 0.8 grams per kg of body weight, which is roughly around 70 grams for an adult woman. Higher levels are required for growing children, during pregnancy and lactation and the older individual. People above the age of 65 seem to do better on 1.2–1.5 grams/kg of body weight, with athletes and those actively trying to gain muscle and bone mass aiming to get around 1.6 grams/kg body weight.

As you transition into menopause, aiming for 1.2–1.5 grams/kg of body weight is probably a good idea, as this is a time when bone loss is maximum. People consuming in excess of 1.6 grams/kg will probably have no advantage and may in fact neglect other important nutrients in their diet, including fibre and other micronutrients.

Whole plant foods are always a better source of protein than protein supplements, as Rohini, a nutritionist, discusses in Chapter 15. Rohini also discusses who may benefit from protein supplements. Plant protein sources are as healthy as animal-derived protein sources, with the added benefit of coming packed with fibre and phytonutrients and without the higher levels of saturated fat.

Fats

Polyunsaturated fats (PUFAs) are important for bone formation by helping improve calcium absorption in the small intestine whereas saturated fats hinder absorption. Extra virgin olive oil, nuts and seeds in one's diet can provide the appropriate amount of PUFA to help with bone metabolism and synthesis.

Carbohydrates

These foods are the main source of energy for our body, and if they come from fruits and vegetables, they seem to be much more bone promoting than if they come from ultra-processed grains. Fruit and vegetables form alkaline precursors, which seem to promote bone formation. They are also anti-inflammatory and can contribute to the healing of microfractures and bone healing. A study from Scotland showed that a fibre-rich diet was associated with better bone density than a nutrient-poor ultra-processed food diet.[1] Prunes are rich in compounds such as phenolics, inositol and vitamin K and seem to be beneficial in post-menopausal women in preserving bone.[2] As they are rich in fibre, prunes also help relieve constipation.

Important micronutrients for bone health

Minerals

Calcium

Calcium has several vital roles in the body as well as making bones and teeth stronger. It is important for muscle and nerve function, with calcium blood levels finely tuned within a narrow safe range. Recommended daily allowances are rather variable all over the world, with the USA recommending over 1000 mg, possibly because of a meat-heavy acidic diet consumed by most Americans, which means calcium excretion and turnover are higher (resulting in higher calcium needs). In the UK, daily calcium recommendations are 700 mg, while some countries do not seem to have a recommended daily allowance.

Calcium comes from the soil

It is important to understand that calcium is a mineral present in soil and therefore most plant foods are rich in this mineral (cows get their calcium from plants too). Most low-oxalate greens (kale, bok choy, watercress, cabbage, collard greens for example), oranges, figs, nuts, seeds, nut butters and legumes are rich sources of calcium. Greens such as spinach and Swiss chard are higher in oxalates, and this can impair calcium absorption from the gut.

Soya foods such as calcium-set tofu and tempeh are also excellent sources of calcium. Choose soya milk and other plant-based milks that are fortified with calcium.

Dairy is also a rich source of calcium but with over 70 per cent of the world's population lactose intolerant with unpleasant symptoms of bloating and gas, it is possible to get all the calcium you need from a plant-based diet.

Calcium supplements are rarely ever required, except if there is a disorder affecting calcium absorption, and studies suggest it may be in fact harmful by suddenly elevating serum calcium levels and disrupting a delicate balance, especially in women post-menopause. I would suggest checking with your doctor before supplementing with calcium. Instead focus on whole plant-based sources, of which there are plenty.

Other minerals

Phosphorus, copper, magnesium, zinc, boron and silicon are all important micronutrients needed in tiny amounts for healthy bone formation. All of these minerals are present in vegetables, nuts and seeds, so eating a diverse and varied plant-predominant diet will meet your needs in most situations.

Vitamin D

Vitamin D functions much more like a hormone as we actually synthesize it in our skin from exposure to sunlight where UV-B rays act on cholesterol to activate formation of the active form of vitamin D.

Vitamin D is important in the absorption of calcium from the gut and in addition to its crucial role in bone formation, vitamin D helps in the formation of 'fast twitch' or type 2 muscle fibres which are helpful in the prevention of falls.

Vitamin D deficiency is common in countries above 30 degree latitudes, such as the UK, especially in the autumn and winter months. Therefore, a vitamin D supplement is the best way to get an optimum serum level of vitamin D (see Chapter 18).

Vitamin B12

This is a vitamin made by microorganisms in the soil and anyone on a plant-based diet as well as all omnivores over the age of 50 (USA guidance) and over 65 (UK guidance) should supplement this in their diet (Chapter 18). B12 deficiency is very serious and can result in falls because of damage to the nerves, resulting in fractures.

Vitamin C

Abundant in fruit and vegetables, a recommended daily dose is available through consuming a single orange. Even so, it seems that a large proportion of the American population has insufficient intakes of this vitamin which helps prevent bone loss by its inhibitory action on bone-clearing osteoclasts and is also a cofactor in the formation of collagen, which is essential to bone formation.

Vitamin K

Vitamin K seems to be important for us to hold on to calcium in the bone whereas vitamin D helps in getting calcium into the blood from our gut. In one study post-menopausal women in Japan seemed to benefit from a vitamin K supplement. More research is awaited in this area. Sauerkraut, kimchi and natto (fermented soya beans) are good sources of vitamin K2, which seems to be the component relevant to bone, but there is no consensus on a daily requirement. Precursors of vitamin K are also present in green leafy vegetables, so consuming these regularly will provide the vitamin K needed for your body.

Vitamin A

Vitamin A is available from carotenoid-rich foods such as colourful fruits and squash, sweet potatoes and carrots. Vitamin A is needed for healthy hair, skin and eyes and has an **antioxidant** effect and is considered to be bone protective. Be cautious of supplementing vitamin A without supervision, as it is toxic in high doses. The safest way is to get your vitamin A from fruits and vegetables.

Food-first approach

Some supplements such as B6 and B12 together were found to reduce bone density in a study and therefore taking multivitamin combinations with large amounts of vitamins unnecessarily without proper advice can be harmful. A food-first approach is advised in most situations, with only certain supplements shown to have proven benefit (Chapter 18).

Body weight and composition

As bones respond to body weight and become stronger, it is important to understand that having too low a BMI is counterproductive and increases the risk of osteoporosis and weaker bones. There are at least four good quality large studies, including a 2023 study from the UK Biobank, confirming **vegetarians** and pescatarians are at higher risk of hip fractures.[3,4] The number of vegans was too small to be studied separately. As these groups tend to be slimmer with lower BMI, it is not surprising that they are at higher risk of osteoporosis. Taking care to include key nutrients through a plant-predominant diet with certain supplements and strength training can reduce these risks. The same studies found that these groups were at lower risks of type 2 diabetes, certain cancers and heart disease, which of course is good news. Carrying excessive body weight or being obese is also harmful as visceral fat in particular is inflammatory and bone production is poor in medically obese individuals, besides the multitude of risks of excess body weight.

On the other hand, muscles are what load our bones, so gaining muscle as we age is really important in prevention of sarcopenia and osteoporosis.

A BMI of around 23 with a high muscle to fat ratio is ideal for bone strength. A body composition DEXA scan, which can give an estimate of lean mass and visceral fat, in addition to bone density, with lifestyle advice from a trained lifestyle medicine professional is helpful for women who wish to change their body composition to lose fat and gain muscle.

For those women doing strength training, which has benefits for all women, creatine monohydrate as a supplement (around 4 grams a day) is very useful in improving workouts as it makes energy readily available to muscle tissue. It is also known to have benefits in cognition. Most other supplements are not recommended and can sometimes be harmful, especially as the supplement industry is poorly regulated, with very little quality control.

Calcium thieves

Alcohol is harmful to bone formation. It may cause this effect by loss of calcium in the urine but also, possibly, by direct toxic effects.

Smoking, excess caffeine consumption, sugar-sweetened beverages, especially fizzy cola drinks which contain salt and phosphoric acid, can result in calcium losses in the urine. In addition, dietary excesses of sodium (main source of salt is in **ultraprocessed foods** including bread, cheese etc.) of even an additional 1 gram daily over a year can result in the loss of 1 per cent of our bone mass. Most people consume far in excess of the WHO recommendation of 5 g of salt (or 2000 mg of sodium) per day, which is less than one level teaspoon per day.

Medications for osteoporosis

Drugs used to treat osteoporosis certainly have a role, and are necessary for people at a high risk of having a fracture. If you need medications to manage your osteoporosis, do ensure you are being guided by a qualified health professional. Irrespective of this, all the dietary and lifestyle factors should still be followed to the best of your ability, to help improve your quality of life.

Menopause mantra: *My bone health is important*

- Bone is living tissue and responds to good nutrition and exercise.
- Osteoporosis is a disease when bones become weak.
- Sarcopenia is the loss of muscle mass and muscle wasting.
- It is never too late to make changes to exercise and diet to manage these conditions.
- Strength and resistance exercises twice a week for 30 minutes each are recommended.
- Resistance bands, body weight exercises, skipping, jumping jacks all count.
- Balance and flexibility exercises are important to help prevent falls.
- Protein is an important macronutrient that is required in building bone and muscle.
- Choose whole-food plant protein sources such as soya products and legumes.
- Calcium, vitamin D and a number of other micronutrients are needed for healthy bones.
- A food-first approach will provide the vast majority of nutrients needed to build bone.
- Vitamin D supplements and vitamin B12 supplements are usually a good idea.
- Supplements of calcium are rarely ever needed and may be harmful.
- Maintain a healthy body weight, and increase muscle mass.
- Avoid alcohol, excess caffeine and smoking.

6

Still in my prime: Menopause and the workplace

Women are living longer and retiring later, more so now than ever before. Periods, perimenopause and menopause affect over half the world's population and yet here we are with women still facing stigma in society when talking about the changes our body goes through.

The workplace is no different, with women all over the world having a similar experience when it comes to menopause, most of it not good. This means women often have to pretend everything's fine and carry on as normal whilst experiencing the many troublesome symptoms of perimenopause and menopause. Painful or heavy periods, chronic pain and fatigue from conditions like endometriosis, anxiety or depression associated with **infertility**, miscarriage, severe premenstrual syndrome, PCOS and other gynaecological conditions can also persist into perimenopause.

Women often do not know where to turn for help, especially if the symptoms of menopause occur much earlier than expected, as they may with POI, early menopause, surgical or medical menopause or if they are in perimenopause years before their periods stop. Women say they often feel dismissed and are hesitant to seek medical advice, especially if they have had a previous negative encounter with a healthcare provider. Most women are also not aware of their rights in workplaces and even if they are, don't want to draw attention to themselves for fear of judgement and losing career opportunities. I can empathize.

Girl power

The average age for women to be working now has increased by 3.9 years to 64.3 years old in 2020 compared to 1986, as per figures from the UK government.[1] The employment rate for 50–64-year-olds is around 72 per cent and for 35–49-year-olds is over 85 per cent, with the female employment rate in the UK 72.3 per cent in the first quarter of 2023.[2] In the USA, female employment rates are lower at 54.7 per cent in 2022. These figures do not even consider the sheer number of women in unpaid employment, caring for their elderly parents, children and partners, with little time for self-care.

With women forming such a huge part of the workforce, how is it that these conversations haven't happened at the highest level until perhaps very recently? Women need workplace policies that are implemented with accessible guidelines firmly in place. After all, menopause is part of working women's lives and should be recognized as such. However, research into menopause and its effects on work and physical and mental wellbeing is lacking for the most part. As a taboo subject, menopause remains unrecognized and unaddressed within an organizational context.[3]

Workplace environment

One would think that doctors with all their knowledge would have been trailblazers, challenging existing culture, talking openly about the effects their menopausal symptoms were having on them and their work. Not so. The situation is not much better for women doctors than it is for other working women.[4]

A British Medical Association survey of 2000 women doctors in 2020 confirmed this workplace narrative is alive and kicking, with many doctors saying they are silent because they are afraid of the repercussions and reactions from managers and colleagues. The survey findings are interesting, with 93 per cent of survey respondents confirming experiencing symptoms as a result of the menopause, and 65 per cent experiencing both physical and mental symptoms. Nine out of ten women said their symptoms had impacted their working lives, with nearly four in ten saying that the impact was significant.[5] These statistics are hugely important and are very similar to my own experience and that of my female colleagues.

The good news is that NHS England has since signed the Menopause Workplace Pledge in June 2022, in a move that demonstrates a commitment to ensuring employees experiencing the menopause feel well informed and supported while at work.[6,7]

We need to do better

A survey of over 4000 women in perimenopause and menopause was published in 2022 by the Fawcett Society commissioned by Channel 4 for a TV documentary titled *Davina McCall: Sex, Mind and the Menopause*. It is the largest survey in the UK of its kind, with the report highlighting that one in ten women who worked during the menopause had left their job due to their symptoms, and eight out of ten women said their employer hadn't shared information, trained staff, or put in place a menopause absence policy. Almost half of women hadn't approached their GPs, with three in ten women seeing delays in diagnosis. Only four in ten women were offered HRT in a timely fashion. The report highlighted the lack of basic support for women in the workplace, with no provision, support networks or policies in place for eight in ten women going through menopause.[8]

Consequences of menopause symptoms on work outcomes

Workplace stigma and the failure to recognize the impact of menopausal symptoms on work means that these attitudes have far reaching consequences for the individual, for the employer, for the country's economic growth and for the morale of other staff.

Women often step down from more senior roles or turn down the promotions which they are due, or hand in their resignations, because of the institutional lack of support and failure to recognize the impact of menopausal symptoms, often resulting in severe stress and burnout.[9] This is a real waste of talent, with employers losing highly skilled individuals who would have continued to be an asset for several more years, if they were given a chance. It is also deeply distressing for the women themselves.

Normalizing menopause at the workplace

The largest study to date, conducted by the Mayo Clinic in the US in 2023, analysed responses from 4400 women aged 45–60 and found nearly 11 per cent reported missing work in the past 12 months due to menopausal symptoms such as hot flushes and night sweats. The study highlighted the need to improve medical treatment and make the workplace environment more supportive for women in menopause. The Mayo Clinic study estimated an annual loss of $1.8 billion in the USA, based on workdays missed due to menopause symptoms, and recommended further research in this area.[10]

People most at risk

In another study from the USA published in 2023 around one-third of women reported moderate to severe difficulties coping at work because of menopausal symptoms.[4] Those with financial difficulties, associated health issues, depression and women who had job insecurity or were unappreciated or dissatisfied with their work seem to be at greatest risk. More awareness is needed, among employers in all sectors, of the effects of perimenopause and menopause on women in these groups.

Employers also need to be aware of the particular challenges in menopause faced by women who may have physical or learning challenges, and those from other minority backgrounds, including people of colour (Chapter 7).

Transgender, non-binary and intersex staff may experience the menopause differently, either due to age-related hormonal changes or hormone treatments and surgery. Managing menopause can be a particular challenge, as some staff may not wish to disclose their menopausal symptoms, as this may mean disclosing their trans or intersex status, for fear of harassment and job loss. It can therefore be particularly difficult for these employees to access support and/ or ask for adjustments, as they may hesitate in coming forward.[11,12,13] Employers should take extra precautions and make provisions to handle these situations sensitively and in complete confidence.

Call to action

A House of Commons Committee report with recommendations to government was submitted in 2022. This was on the back of the findings of a 2019 survey by the Chartered Institute of Personnel and Development (CIPD)[14,15] that three in five women aged 45–55 were negatively affected at work, with around 900,000 women in the UK leaving their jobs over an undefined period of time because of menopausal symptoms.

Menopause discrimination is largely covered under the Equality Act (2010), under three protected characteristics: age, sex and disability discrimination.

Things are changing for the better in the UK but at a pace that is still doing a disservice to many women.

Leading from the front

There are several steps that any employer can and should take, preferably enforced by the government. Workplace menopause education should be for employers and employees of all genders, so women can be supported through this often difficult transition, so they can continue to be valuable and appreciated members of the workforce. Flexible working policies can also make a huge difference.

Challenging prevailing attitudes from the top down and signposting to the right resources can be brought in by even small employers to support women through menopause, as well as allowing for unscheduled breaks, and providing simple amenities such as a fan, cold water, a seat near a window and toilet facilities.

For bigger employers, introducing and embedding workplace menopause policies within occupational health and safety and health promotion policies that are openly discussed and shared to provide support rather than gathering dust in the corner of an office should be mandatory. Having a person who women can approach in confidence, usually known as a Menopause Champion, allowing for menopause or menstrual leave without repercussions on career progress and having regular educational updates and staff briefings can go a long way in both staff retention and improving staff morale.[13]

Menopause mantra: *I know my rights*

- Older women form a large part of the workforce all over the world.
- Menopause stigma both in society and in the workplace is real.
- Normalizing conversations around menopause is important to break the taboo.
- More severe symptoms are associated with worse work outcomes: leaving one's job, missing workdays, turning down senior roles.
- Certain groups are at risk from work pressures in menopause: those with financial or health difficulties, those facing physical and learning challenges, and minority groups.
- Workplace menopause education needs to happen with all employees by all employers, enforced by the government's menopause policies.
- Support and flexible working options should be available to women who need them.
- Simple adjustments to the workplace, such as flexible working, improving room ventilation, toilet facilities, drinking water and rest breaks, can make a difference.
- Developing an inclusive culture to allow open conversations about menopause.

7

From the fringe: Menopause experience in minority groups

The way women experience perimenopause and menopause all over the world can vary widely. My observation from my own clinical practice is that every woman has her own menopause story and is unique in the way she experiences and deals with menopause. There are, however, particular challenges faced by certain groups of people that may make their menopause transition harder than usual.

A lack of awareness and failure to recognize these differences amongst health professionals can make it more difficult for women from these backgrounds to access care. Research in these groups is particularly scarce despite the knowledge that there are many differences in symptom reporting and uptake of health services. Some of this chapter may make for upsetting reading, but it is information worth knowing and sharing.

Racial differences in onset of natural menopause

The age of natural menopause is around 51.4 years around the world, but the range can vary between ages 45–55. On closer examination, women from certain parts of the world may experience menopause earlier or later. For example, South Asian women may go through menopause a few years earlier, around the age of 47. This is important information for women and health professionals, as women from these groups may experience perimenopause earlier. There also seems to be a higher incidence of POI and early menopause in countries with a medium or low Human Development Index.

Black women can experience menopause up to two years earlier than their white counterparts and studies suggest that their perimenopause and menopause symptoms are often more intense and last longer.

Black and East Asian women are at much higher risk of heart disease, type 2 diabetes, hypertension and other chronic illnesses. Bone mineral density is lowest in Asians, and highest in African-American women who have a reduced risk of osteoporosis. Black women who are medically obese or overweight with metabolic abnormalities are particularly at higher risk of heart disease in perimenopause and menopause.[1]

If women and health professionals are not aware of these variations, women may miss receiving timely care for their menopausal symptoms, both in the short term but also in the longer term (bone, brain and heart health).

If you are a woman of colour, there is no reason to ever be denied HRT by a health professional based on your race and ethnicity, as is known to happen. Instead, the decision to prescribe HRT or any other medication must always be taken on an individual basis.

It is also helpful to be aware of certain ethnic variations, as doses may have to be adjusted, with Asian women having significantly higher serum oestradiol levels during treatment with transdermal oestrogen compared with white women, while there may be lower absorption of HRT through the skin (transdermal patches and gel) in Black women when compared with white women, due to differences in skin structure.[2,3,4]

Barriers for people of colour

Cultural and traditional beliefs may make the menopause experience different for many women from certain communities. In a country that is as diverse as the UK (14.4 per cent from the Office for National Statistics in 2019 were from ethnic minority backgrounds, with 46.2 per cent of London residents identifying as Asian, Black, mixed or 'other' ethnic groups), health professionals need to be aware of these differences in the women they see, offering medical and lifestyle advice sensitively and appropriately.[5]

The approach to menopause can also vary widely, with some women accepting this as part of life and putting up with troublesome symptoms, relieved to have periods and childbearing out of the way. In fact, in societies where ageing is accepted and older people are valued, menopause may be welcome, as it can bring power and more equality with men. For others, it might be the opposite, a feeling of no longer being considered a productive member of society, or grief over the perceived loss of femininity. These varying attitudes may also affect a woman's decision about commencing HRT.

A UK study found British South Asian women's experience of hot flushes is more similar to the British white women compared to women in Delhi, India, who did not report hot flushes. However, British South Asians and women in Delhi both reported more weight gain, anxiety, palpitations, joint pains, while white British women had more night sweats, tiredness and were more likely to talk about sexual health.[6]

Immigrants from the Asian subcontinent and Africa, especially first-generation immigrants, may struggle to express their symptoms, and are at risk of getting dismissed by their doctor or prescribed inappropriate medications. Language barrier or cultural hesitancy in sharing private information with friends and family, with a male partner or with male practitioners can also be issues in being heard and receiving care.

Structural racism

A shorter average lifespan for minority groups is said to be linked to 'weathering' or accelerated health declines, due to systemic marginalization. Long-standing gender and racial discrimination, social and economic factors may be responsible for chronic stress and the longer duration and intensity of menopause symptoms in African Caribbean women.[7]

One of the hallmark USA studies of menopause is the Study of Women's Health Across the Nation (SWAN), a multi-site, multi-racial/ ethnic cohort of women, who were enrolled in 1996 at the age of 42 to 52 years and followed for over 25 years, as participants transitioned from pre-menopause through menopause and into early old age.[8]

A 2023 review paper looking at the SWAN study found that systematic exclusion at the start of the study masked the finding that Black and Hispanic women are likely to experience menopause measurably earlier, as well as more intense hot flushes and other menopausal symptoms, when compared to their white counterparts, with discrimination playing a possible role.[9] Black women were twice as likely as white women to have had their womb or ovaries removed, and therefore were half as likely to experience natural menopause – 30 per cent, compared with 15 per cent. Women from marginalized groups are also less likely to be offered HRT compared to other groups.

A mistrust of healthcare systems arising from historical mistreatment and experimentation in Black communities may also make Black women wary of taking HRT, when it could be transformative for that particular individual.

Socio-economic and education status

Many members of these minority groups may be from lower socio-economic or lower education backgrounds, where healthcare is often already compromised. Women who face financial difficulties are more likely to experience worse menopausal symptoms, and are less likely to seek help. A UK study in 2020 found doctors were 29 per cent less likely to prescribe HRT in the most deprived sectors in comparison to the most affluent, with a preference for oral over the more commonly used transdermal HRT preparations.[10]

The importance of diet and lifestyle factors in menopausal symptoms may not be disseminated or stressed enough in these groups, where in fact they would be most beneficial.

Women may find it particularly hard to find the time and financial resources, as well as support within their network, for self-care. Time and effort spent by the government, local council and healthcare teams to support these women, as well as ensuring appropriate resources in multiple languages to educate and dispel commonly held myths, can have a positive impact on menopausal health.

People with disabilities

People with physical or learning disabilities often find they are invisible to not just the rest of the public but also health and social services when it comes to getting the same attention available to able-bodied people. Women with physical hindrances may have difficulty with access to toilets, which may be needed more frequently, for example, with heavy or frequent periods in perimenopause or urinary or bowel frequency in menopause. They may also struggle to access healthcare as they may have visual, hearing or mobility issues.

Women with learning disabilities, and in particular women with Down's syndrome, tend to have an earlier menopause than other women and may also have a poorer understanding of menopause. Epileptic seizures are common in people with learning disabilities, who may experience an increase in seizures in perimenopause and fewer in menopause once hormone levels stabilize.[11] Carers often say they are not trained to recognize symptoms and support these women through menopause.

When dealing with women with learning disabilities, health professionals should remember to lead with open questions in a sensitive manner, as some adults may feel embarrassed to discuss issues around reproductive health and menopause, respecting their privacy and autonomy in decision making when they are their own legal guardians, and also offer the opportunity for discussion in a safe space even when they are not their own legal guardian.[12]

Even if individuals with disabilities do not have a significantly different experience of menopause from other women, there may be issues of accelerated bone loss for those who have mobility impairment, as well as increased risk of cognitive decline or heart disease. Hormone replacement therapy has both greater potential benefits and risks in these groups. Some women may also struggle to remember to take the right dose at the right time. A knowledgeable, empathetic healthcare team is invaluable in these situations.

Multigender experience of menopause

There is very little research on the menopause experienced by the LGBTQIA+ community or the trans community.

Those assigned female at birth including LGBTQIA+, trans, non-binary and intersex people who identify differently from the standard societal expectations, may find it hard to be part of a menopause conversation that talks about only cisgender women, and usually women in heterosexual relationships.

Transgender (as opposed to cisgender) is an umbrella term used to describe 'people whose gender identity, expression, or behaviour is different from those typically associated with their assigned sex at birth'. Trans men may experience symptoms of menopause, even if they are having hormonal treatments or awaiting gender reassignment surgery. Gender-affirming hormone therapy (GAHT) such as testosterone will stop periods but will also cause some of the other effects associated with menopause, including hot flushes, hair loss and vaginal atrophy. Transdermal oestrogen may help with some of these symptoms without impacting transition. Gender dysphoria can also be a real issue for an individual, when having to confront symptoms associated with the female reproductive system while identifying as a man or as non-binary.

Menopausal symptoms such as hot flushes can also be experienced by trans women if levels of oestrogen drop. The doses of oestrogen needed in the older trans women haven't been clearly worked out yet, and there isn't yet a target goal for hormone levels in trans women over 50.[13] Older trans women who use hormone replacement therapy are at a higher risk than cisgender women of developing stroke, blood clots and other cardiovascular issues.[14]

Being inclusive

The lack of acknowledgement by society and health professionals that menopause can be experienced by genders other than cis women appears to impact the experience of menopause for people who identify differently. Lack of inclusive language and limited understanding often result in people staying away from healthcare, or not wishing to disclose personal information about their gender status, especially in the workplace. This in turn means missing out on the support available to others. Discrimination and harassment are evident not just in the workplace and in broader society but also when seeing a health professional, with many as a result avoiding important interventions, such as cervical screening.

Call to action

In conclusion, there is an urgent need for targeted research into menopause in the groups discussed above, and for increasing awareness and education with appropriate information resources and changes in policies, to help women and those assigned female at birth prepare for the menopause and improve their quality of life.

Health professionals should learn to recognize menopausal symptoms and join the dots, approaching those from diverse backgrounds with sensitivity, acknowledging cultural differences where appropriate, and providing timely lifestyle and medical advice and guidance.

Empowering women

If you belong to one or more of these groups, educating yourself both with the resources available and your rights will allow you to have a better experience of menopause. You may even feel empowered to consider opening up the menopause discussion in your community or group. Please check out the resources at the back of this book.

Menopause mantra: *I will insist on inclusive language*

- Opening up conversations in menopause to include people from minority groups will improve the experience of menopause for all in society.
- There are racial and cultural differences in natural menopause and how menopause is experienced.
- Structural racism has damaging consequences for Black women who may experience more intense menopause symptoms and for longer duration.
- Be aware to ask for resources to suit your special needs – language, audio visual etc.
- People with physical and learning disabilities may be at a particular disadvantage.
- Use inclusive language as menopause can be experienced by anyone who is assigned female at birth.
- Be curious without being intrusive or insensitive when enquiring about someone's menopause experience.

8

The 21st-century woman: Fertility, contraception, infections

Fertility

> 'I thought I had more time. I keep fit, eat well and do not smoke or drink alcohol.'

Case: Debbie, my 39-year-old patient, was having a few missed cycles, mood changes and occasional hot flushes, which she had put down initially to stress. After a thorough medical assessment, I attributed her symptoms to perimenopause.

A woman may start noticing symptoms between two to eight years before periods completely stop, with the final menstrual period or menopause marking the end of natural reproduction. As the normal range for menopause is 45–55 years, this can mean a woman may be as young as 37 when she starts to experience perimenopause, with a significantly reduced chance of conceiving spontaneously.

Women who receive a diagnosis of POI before the age of 40 (see Chapter 1) often have not even started thinking of having children. For many women, the perimenopause and menopause can come with a great sense of loss of their youth, femininity and fertility.

Fertility declines steeply with age

The average life expectancy has dramatically increased in the last century, with women in high-income countries living into their 80s with the help of improved sanitation, clean water, vaccinations, modern medicines and better nutrition.

Many women, including my patients in their late 30s, 40s and 50s, look and feel fitter than they did in their 20s, and are in better shape than previous generations. These women are often at the peak of their careers and have deferred starting or completing their family, as they are either not in a relationship or thought they had more time. Women in higher-income countries have been delaying childbirth to at least age 30, as per statistics in 2017, while before the 1960s, women in the US were having their first child around the age of 21.

However, what women often do not know is that the age at which women go through the menopause has not really changed over the years, and neither has the age when the number and quality of the eggs within the ovaries start to decline.

A decline in fertility is seen after the age of 35, and particularly after 37 years in the majority of women. It can be earlier for some and later for others, depending on a number of factors such as genetics, age at which one's mother went through the menopause, co-existing conditions such as endometriosis, adenomyosis, fibroids, PCOS, lifestyle factors such as body weight and smoking. Apart from a reduction in the ability to conceive (**infertility** or **subfertility**) with age, there are other pregnancy-related complications such as increased rates of miscarriage, preterm births, gestational diabetes, congenital malformations and operative deliveries, especially after the age of 40.

Age remains the single most important factor determining ovarian egg reserve and fertility for women, even today in a world of medical advances. There is no known way yet to slow or reverse this decline in the number of eggs.

My patients tell me they are not aware of this rapid age-related fertility decline, especially as they regularly see celebrities announcing pregnancies in their late 40s and 50s, and many of their friends in their late 30s having no apparent difficulty in conceiving.

Assisted reproductive techniques (ART)

Assisted conception techniques such as in vitro fertilization (IVF), intra-uterine insemination (IUI), egg freezing, donor eggs/sperm and surrogacy are often not talked about openly, so women do not always disclose such information despite benefiting from these modern medical advances for fear of being judged by society and even by friends and family. I completely understand their hesitation. Increasingly, more stories are being shared. We heard about Michelle Obama's IVF struggles when her book *Becoming* was published in 2018, helping open up real conversations around fertility.

As a society, we need to do so much more to normalize conversations around fertility, encouraging choice and autonomy, as well as all available options to build a family. As well as normalizing the choice not to have children either.

Women in their late 20s and 30s who I speak to in public forums have all heard of the biological clock, but do not think it applies to them until much later. The irony is that career progression and family building are directly at loggerheads with each other in many industries, leaving women frustrated as they sometimes have to choose between the two. Finding a suitable partner or the finances to do fertility preservation techniques, such as egg freezing, or the support to have a child when single, are just some of the challenges faced by women.

Education about the female reproductive system and increasing awareness about age-related and lifestyle-related fertility decline is important as are honest conversations about the true success of fertility-preserving options, so women are fully informed from an early age.

Helping yourself

Educate yourself as early as possible about the age-related decline in fertility and see a recommended fertility specialist if you envisage your own biological children in the future. You can then be advised about your options, including egg and embryo freezing after a thorough medical history to check if you have gynaecological conditions that may compromise fertility, such as fibroids, PCOS, endometriosis and adenomyosis. You may consider having your ovarian egg reserve checked through blood tests such as AMH (anti-Mullerian hormone) and a pelvic ultrasound scan, so you can make an informed decision. While egg freezing techniques have come a long way, the overall success of artificial reproductive technology is still lower than women believe, so it is important to factor this in when making your decisions.

Do use the advice from the lifestyle pillars chapters to optimize your lifestyle and nutrition, avoiding tobacco, alcohol and drugs that can harm your ovaries and your fertility.

If you find yourself in the same situation as my patient at the beginning of this chapter, do remember there are several ways of expanding a family not involving one's own genetic material, whether it is through egg donation, adoption or fostering. Debbie was advised to use an egg donor after detailed discussions with a fertility specialist. You may wish to seek the help of a fertility therapist to help you work through your feelings of loss and grief. I wish you the very best.

Menopause mantra: *I will consider my fertility options sooner rather than later*

- A decline in fertility is seen from 35, and particularly after 37 years in most women.
- You are born with a fixed number of eggs in your ovaries.
- Age remains the single most important factor determining ovarian egg reserve and fertility.
- There is no known way to slow or reverse this decline in the number of eggs (oocytes).
- Address lifestyle factors early: body weight, smoking, alcohol.
- Address conditions such as painful periods, PCOS, endometriosis, adenomyosis, fibroids.
- See a reputed fertility specialist early to assess your ovarian egg reserve and your options.
- Assisted reproductive technology (ART) such as in vitro fertilization (IVF), intra-uterine insemination (IUI), egg freezing, donor eggs/sperm and surrogacy may need to be considered.
- Consider ART fertility-preserving options, such as egg and embryo freezing, but be aware success rates are not as high as many think.
- Remember there are many other non-conventional ways to build a family.

Contraception in perimenopause and menopause

Case: 'Nothing. Surely I cannot get pregnant at my age,' stated Laura, my 47-year-old patient, when I asked her what contraception she was currently using.

It is not uncommon for many women to be confused about contraception as they approach menopause. As ovulatory cycles become fewer in perimenopause, pregnancy becomes much less likely. Women are still potentially fertile in their 40s, even though pregnancy is more likely to end in a miscarriage and with higher maternal and foetal complications.

It is important to have time to think about your contraceptive options, and base your decision on your past experience and your preference, but also on scientific expert guidance, rather than hearsay, as there is a lot of misinformation about the reliable contraception methods that I discuss here.

Medical contraceptive advice

You should use effective contraception each time you have vaginal sex with a man to avoid unintended pregnancy, for at least two years after your last period if your periods have completely stopped before the age of 50.

If you are above the age of 50 years, it is recommended to use reliable contraception every time you have vaginal sex with a man for one year after your last menstrual period. This is also the advice if you are on hormone replacement therapy. HRT is not a form of contraception.

If your periods have stopped for any other reason, if your bleeding patterns suddenly change, if you are on hormonal contraception, or if you are unsure, you should always consult your doctor for further advice.

Which is the best contraception in perimenopause?

All contraceptive options may be appropriate during perimenopause and no method is contraindicated based on age alone. After a thorough discussion about all available options, a detailed medical history and examination and a woman's preference, fitting a levonorgestrel intrauterine device (IUS or intrauterine system) allows for both highly effective contraception and management of heavy periods, endometriosis or adenomyosis if these are issues in perimenopause. The IUS can be left in place for a number of years, as instructed by the manufacturer. This hormone-containing coil can also provide the progesterone arm of HRT (along with an oestrogen patch or gel) for a number of years from the time it is fitted (as per manufacturer licence), if hormone replacement is indicated.

Other contraceptive methods

You may also decide to opt for sterilization, a permanent option, and this could be either you or your partner opting for a vasectomy, the latter a much more straightforward procedure.

The Pill (COCP) or combined hormonal contraceptive pill can be used in the absence of contraindications until the age of 50. The Pill has the added benefit of relieving perimenopausal symptoms, managing irregular periods, improving acne, protecting bones and reducing the risk of ovarian, bowel and endometrial cancers. The low-dose COCP that is used nowadays can be taken back-to-back without monthly breaks, as there is no medical reason to have a monthly withdrawal bleed, and will give better control of perimenopausal symptoms.

Perimenopausal women should not use oestrogen-containing contraceptives if they smoke or have a history of oestrogen-dependent cancer, heart disease, high blood pressure, diabetes or blood clots.

Progesterone-only contraception (pill, implant, depot) can be taken on its own or in combination with oestrogen replacement therapy, if there is a need to address both perimenopausal symptoms and contraception.

Non-hormonal options such as the copper IUD and barrier methods, including male and female condoms, cervical cap and diaphragm, are available for those wishing to avoid hormonal methods. The condom has the added benefit of protection against sexually transmitted infections (STIs).

Fertility awareness is rarely used correctly, and is thus not a reliable method of contraception, and the withdrawal method is even more unreliable. Natural family planning methods can be unpredictable, particularly in the perimenopause when a woman's regular menstrual pattern usually changes.

Emergency contraception

There is no upper age limit for emergency contraception, which is indicated for any woman who still needs contraception who has had unprotected sex or contraceptive failure (a split condom or missed pills). The emergency IUD is the more effective method compared to pills and has the advantage that it can remain in place for ongoing contraception.

Stopping contraception

Women can stop using contraception at the age of 55, if they are still having periods, as getting pregnant naturally after this is very rare, although decisions are best made on an individual basis.

It is sensible to use a barrier method, such as condoms, in new relationships to avoid getting STIs, even after the menopause.

The UK Faculty of Sexual and Reproductive Healthcare recommends that women aged 50 years and older using a progestogen-only method who have not had periods for 12 months can have their FSH levels measured on two occasions, at least six weeks apart; if both are greater than or equal to 30 IU/L then contraception is only required for a further 12 months.[1]

Menopause mantra: *I will use effective protection to avoid unintended pregnancy*

- Use reliable contraception for one year after the last menstrual period if above the age of 50 and for two years if periods stop below the age of 50.
- HRT is not contraception.
- No contraceptive method is contraindicated based on age alone.
- Informed decisions based on evidence and preference are important.
- The hormone-containing intra-uterine system can have several benefits in perimenopause.
- Fertility awareness methods and withdrawal methods are unreliable.
- Women still having periods can stop using contraception after age 55.
- Seek reliable contraceptive advice.

Sexually transmitted infections (STIs) in perimenopause and menopause

There appears to be a lack of knowledge of STIs and safer sex among many older women. They are also less likely to use barrier protection, as pregnancy is usually no longer a concern.

Common infections

Chlamydia, gonorrhoea, trichomonas vaginalis, genital warts caused by human papillomavirus (HPV), herpes are the common STIs (sexually transmitted infections) you may have heard of. More serious STIs include Hepatitis B and C, syphilis and HIV (human immunodeficiency virus).

More so now than ever before, women continue to be sexually active in perimenopause and after menopause. Women are often not aware of the importance of using barrier protection such as male or female condoms and dental dams for oral sex, especially in new sexual encounters where partners have not had an STI screen for common infections.

Cervical screening

Current cervical screening to detect abnormal precancer cells and strains of HPV responsible for causing cervical cancer stops at 64 years on the NHS UK cervical screening programme, unless there is a medical indication to continue. It is important to keep your appointment when invited for cervical screening, usually every five years after the age of 50.

The HPV vaccine is offered to schoolgirls and boys and to women until age 25 on the NHS to reduce the risk of cervical cancer. Although women can have the vaccine until the age of 45, HPV vaccination is less likely to offer benefit at this point in life, given that most adults over 25 will already have been infected with HPV. There's no reliable routine test or screening programme to check for high-risk HPV infections in men.

Raising awareness in older women

During perimenopause and menopause, it is still possible to contract STIs through unprotected sexual contact, including oral, anal and vaginal sex.

Vaginal atrophy or thinning of the skin due to low levels of oestrogen increases the chance of tears, making it easier and increasing the risk of HIV transmission during vaginal sex as well as common vaginal infections (not STIs) such as bacterial vaginosis and thrush (vulvovaginal candidiasis).

Consider using vaginal oestrogen regularly as it is safe for the vast majority of women, after discussion with your doctor. It can help make the vagina more resistant to infections.

Always use barrier protection

Using condoms will protect a woman from most STIs by about 98 per cent.

A recent study from Australia, looking at trends between 2000 and 2018, found that STIs (chlamydia and gonorrhoea) are increasing at a faster rate among older women than among younger women.[2] Although there is more of a concern with STIs in younger women, STIs from unprotected sexual intercourse are still an issue for older women, causing unwanted side effects of vaginal discharge, pelvic pain, bleeding and sometimes systemic disease with the more serious infections.

Women and clinicians may underestimate the risk of infection, so a proper risk assessment should be undertaken. Do bring it to the notice of your health professional if you think you are at risk of an STI or have non-specific vulval or vaginal symptoms such as irritation, which may be mistaken for a symptom of menopause.

Menopause manta: *Use barrier protection to avoid STIs*

- Menopause and older age are not a protection against sexually transmitted infections (STIs).
- Chlamydia is the most commonly reported STI.
- Get tested and ask for partner/s to be tested for common STIs even before having sex.
- Always use condoms and dental dams to practise safer sex to avoid STIs.
- Using vaginal oestrogen can help prevent vaginal tears and reduce the risk of infections.

PART TWO

AGE-PROOF YOUR MENOPAUSE – THE POWER OF LIFESTYLE

Society, public health policies and the medical community have all uniformly neglected to recognize women are different from men in myriad ways. This has resulted in health and workplace policies that do not always serve our best interests, whatever our age or stage of life.

In this section, I am excited to share lifestyle advice based on science, as well as my decades of clinical experience in obstetrics and gynaecology, to help you prepare for perimenopause and menopause with confidence. This is information I wish I had had access to decades ago.

By applying the six pillars of lifestyle medicine, you will age-proof your perimenopausal years and menopausal decades to help you live your best life. You will learn the principles of lifestyle medicine and its six pillars that we know great health is based on, adding years to your life and more importantly, life to your years. You deserve no less.

I will help you understand the vital role of physical movement and exercise in this important phase of your life, the impact of fluctuating hormones on sleep, the effect of stress on menopausal symptoms and how nurturing positive social connections can significantly influence your experience of menopause. As well as focusing on the scientific evidence of the benefits of a plant-predominant way of eating in menopause, you will learn about the true effects of substances like alcohol and tobacco on your menopausal symptoms.

By the end of this part, you will feel empowered to make a positive difference to your life.

9

Lifestyle matters: The six pillars of lifestyle medicine

Even as a doctor who trained for over a decade in obstetrics and gynaecology in two different continents, I had no idea where to access reliable lifestyle information that could help me when I needed it most. As doctors, we were not taught at any point in our careers that the food we eat, or our lifestyle, have a major role to play in illness or health. This is changing in the medical world, although at a slow pace.

Every aspect of our health, from birth until the very end, can benefit from good nutrition and a healthy lifestyle. It is not lack of motivation or self-control that has created the current health crisis and a society that is sicker by the day. Most of us have not been taught or equipped with the right tools to build positive habits. The issue is much wider and at a much higher level than us. However, as individuals we should not throw our hands in the air and resign ourselves to ill health, once we have the information that can change our lives for the better.

Health span, not life span

Of the top ten causes of death in the world, you may be surprised to know that seven of them are preventable non-communicable diseases such as heart disease, stroke, type 2 diabetes, cancer and dementia. Most of us will know of at least one person in our close network with one or more of these conditions. Two-thirds of adults aged over 65 are expected to be living with multiple health conditions by 2035, with 17 per cent living with four or more diseases, double the number in 2015.[1] One-third of these people would have a neurological condition like dementia or a mental illness like depression.[2] This is a serious health crisis.

Healthcare professionals, including myself, see this daily in our clinical practice. Most of our patients, in fact upwards of eight out of ten, suffer from **chronic illnesses** that are lifestyle-related.

Women's health is no exception, with coronary heart disease being the single biggest killer of women worldwide. Oestrogen is protective, so women tend to develop heart disease later in life in the post-menopausal decades. Symptoms of heart disease can differ in women from men, for example, chest discomfort, jaw pain, feeling sick, sweaty, lightheaded, bouts of coughing, and even feelings of anxiety. Women are often dismissed with their symptoms ignored, even in emergency departments, often with disastrous consequences.

There are many conditions that also put women at increased risk of heart disease later in life, that you may not be aware of. These include endometriosis, PCOS, miscarriages, raised blood pressure or diabetes in pregnancy and infertility, but there is little awareness of this, both by public health and the medical community. A lot can be done to prevent heart disease at a much earlier stage. Another missed opportunity to help women.

Certain cancers such as breast, bowel, ovarian and womb, as well as hip fractures from osteoporosis, also contribute to mortality (death rates) and morbidity (suffering) in women as they get older (see Chapter 13).

In 2019, the World Health Organization (WHO) declared **Alzheimer's disease** and other forms of dementia as the seventh leading cause of death globally, disproportionately affecting women. Alzheimer's disease, a form of dementia, is now the leading cause of death in women in the UK.[3,4]

Dementia is a heart-breaking condition affecting memory and cognition, often resulting in losing one's identity, and not being able to recognize loved ones. None of us wants ourselves or our loved ones to ever be diagnosed with dementia. There are many ways for women to build cognitive resilience and cognitive reserve to reduce our risk of dementia, using lifestyle modifications. We need to develop habits that grow our brain, and improve brain health through exercise, learning a new language, new hobbies and by avoiding isolation by actively participating in community activities when we are still in good health.

Defining lifestyle medicine

You may have never heard of a medical specialty called **lifestyle medicine**. Most doctors haven't heard of it either. Many of the principles of lifestyle medicine have been practised since the time of

Hippocrates, a Greek physician, widely considered the father of modern medicine for his revolutionary approach to health and illness. Today, lifestyle medicine as we know it is a fairly new discipline that runs alongside Western medicine, and is fast gaining popularity.

Lifestyle medicine, as defined by the American College of Lifestyle Medicine (ACLM), is the use of evidence-based lifestyle approaches for the treatment, prevention and sometimes reversal of lifestyle-related chronic disease.[5] Self-care and self-management are at its heart, allowing you to be in the driving seat rather than your treating doctor.

In lifestyle medicine, you are involved in making informed decisions about your health every step of the way. Lifestyle medicine walks alongside Western medicine. It is not one or the other. Lifestyle medicine is not complementary or alternative medicine or functional medicine, although it may work alongside these disciplines.

Making behaviour and lifestyle changes can go a very long way in reducing chronic diseases and achieving optimal health, both in the short term and longer term, helping you to avoid unnecessary medications or surgery or significantly reducing the need for them. These changes are most valuable when adopted in early in life where possible, and are perhaps even more important as one heads towards menopause and older age.

Living longer, living better

Educate yourself to make informed health choices when faced with menopause or with a health problem. Rather than feeling overwhelmed or disempowered, which sometimes happens when a doctor advises only medications or surgery, applying evidence-based lifestyle medicine principles alongside Western medical treatment as needed can be extremely empowering. My advice to anyone reading this book is to make changes to the best of your ability, whether you are in midlife or not even close.

Chain reaction

Starting with one aspect of lifestyle tends to have a positive effect on the other aspects of one's life. When you sleep better, you tend to stress less, make better food and drink choices and exercise more. A domino effect or chain reaction is set off.

There are six pillars of lifestyle medicine that can help you optimize health. I suggest you bring a few simple achievable changes to your lifestyle initially, which you can build on over time. To reduce menopause symptoms such as disturbed sleep, simple changes such as ensuring a regular bedtime routine, going for a walk outdoors, eating your evening meal early, or doing a simple workout daily are usually achievable. Do it without judgement, so you enjoy the transition.

In the chapters that follow, I will discuss how each of these six lifestyle pillars can help you manage your perimenopause and menopause symptoms now and in the years to come.

The six pillars of lifestyle medicine

1. A predominantly whole-food, plant-based diet.
2. Regular physical activity.
3. Restorative sleep.
4. Stress management.
5. Avoidance of risky substances.
6. Positive social connections.

Menopause mantra: *I want to live better, not just longer*

- Menopausal health will benefit from good nutrition and healthy lifestyle.
- It's never too early or too late to make lifestyle changes.
- Make changes in any one area of lifestyle and other areas will follow.
- Make small changes and build up slowly, until the change becomes a habit.
- Enjoy the transition, making changes without judgement.
- Educate yourself using reliable health sources.

10

Food for thought: Nourishing your body through menopause

Nutrition is the lifestyle pillar that is the most contentious yet probably the most powerful of the six lifestyle pillars that all health is based on. Our relationship with food is complex, and is closely entwined with habit, culture and childhood memories. Many people now recognize, especially since the start of the pandemic, that neither human health nor planetary health can sustain our current way of eating. This next section is one where my hope is to help you modify your diet forever based on evidence, choosing a sustainable, nutritious and delicious way of eating that is kind to your body as well as to the planet we inhabit.

What we eat on a daily basis is the one aspect of our lives that we can control to a large extent as adults, and is also the one most amenable to change, with positive results for many health measurements and body weight seen in a matter of weeks.

Why is it, then, that we are facing a global health crisis with 52 per cent of the world's population now either overweight or obese?[1] This is set to rise in the coming years. Closer to home, the figures are even more worrying. The Health Survey for England, published in December 2022, recorded that nearly 60 per cent of women, that is six in ten women, and nearly 70 per cent of men are either overweight or obese. People aged 45–74 are most likely to be overweight or obese.[2] That is the group that includes women in perimenopause and menopause. Excess weight comes with increased health risks and is second only to smoking in causing health problems.

Pervasive misinformation, government policies that subsidise ultraprocessed highly refined foods and animal products, lack of nutrition education, low socio-economic status, the cost of living crisis, and lack of access and education are just some of the factors preventing many people from filling their plates with affordable nutritious food.

The Global Burden of Disease study is the most comprehensive worldwide study to date, tracking 195 countries in their trends in consumption of 15 dietary factors from 1990 to 2017. The study concluded more deaths and disabilities were caused by unhealthy diets, with too low an intake of foods such as whole grains, fruit, vegetables, nuts and seeds, than by any other factors. Cardiovascular disease was the leading cause of diet-related deaths and disability.[3]

In the UK, over half of the British diet now consists of ultra-processed foods (56 per cent) and less than a third (only 28 per cent) of adults were eating the recommended five portions of fruit and vegetables per day in 2018, with eight in ten children not reaching their daily target.[4]

While there is no one diet that experts agree is the best for health or for women around menopause, there is widespread agreement that a diet that is plant predominant, meaning a diet rich in whole plant foods such as fruits, vegetables, wholegrains and legumes, is the one that is consistently associated with good health.

Many of us seem to have lost the ability to listen to the cues our body gives us. We underestimate how intimately our mind is connected to our physical body, often ignoring the signals our body sends us throughout the day. We become vulnerable to misinformation and false promises, especially when it comes to our dietary choices. There are no good foods or bad foods or superfoods that will make or break our health. It is the entire dietary pattern, and how we live our life on a daily basis, that really matters for true wellbeing.

Take the time to educate and empower yourself. Now is as good a time as any other to stop yo-yo dieting, address health issues and live the life you deserve, whether you are pre-menopausal, or in the perimenopausal or post-menopausal phase of life. Better health makes it easier to handle all the other stresses of life.

> If you don't make time for your wellness, you will have to make time for your illness.

This information is not meant to scare you, but instead to empower you. What we choose to put in our mouths every day, and how we live our life, can make a significant difference in dodging the genetic cards we have been dealt in life. Genes are not always our destiny. The statement below, adopted by many health professionals over the years, resonates strongly with me.

'Genetics loads the gun, but lifestyle (diet) pulls the trigger.'[5,6]

11

Diversity of plants: The role of nutrition

I grew up eating the most delicious home cooked South Indian vegetarian food. Amma, my mother had a busy job in senior school as an English and History teacher, while holding down two other jobs as a translator and giving after school tuition. She however, had to find the time to cook for three ravenous children. My dad, an engineer by profession, did all the grocery shopping as it was normal for men to go to the market in Kolkata, unlike in other parts of India.

I complained nonstop that I was eating chapattis (Indian flatbread), sabjis (curried vegetables) and dal or a South Indian breakfast of idlis, fresh coconut chutney and spicy sambhar (fermented steamed rice cakes with savoury lentils) and fresh seasonal fruit for breakfast, while my friends got to enjoy toast with butter or cereal with milk.

Dairy milk, ghee (clarified butter), butter and cooking oils were expensive and rationed out to us, which meant we were eating a plant-predominant diet, rich in whole or **minimally processed** plant foods. My mother, of course, was having none of my complaining, simply pointing out that I was very tall for my age and on the interschool track and basketball teams on this diet, so it must be very good for me. She was of course right, as mothers usually are.

I ate some meat, mostly chicken a few times a year as a teenager and in medical school, but returned to being completely vegetarian (not even eggs) when I was pregnant with our daughters. Once we moved to the UK when I was pregnant with our second daughter, my diet became particularly heavy with dairy products such as cheese, yoghurt, milk (and milk chocolate). There were few meat-free options 30 years ago. I did not realize how much dairy I was consuming until nearly a decade later, when I replaced all dairy with soya products. I had joined my daughters in becoming vegan, to support them in their decision, a year or so after my menopause diagnosis of POI at age 38 and – surprisingly – I felt so much better in myself. It still took me another decade to make the connection between what I ate and my health.

In those days, there were few or no vegan options, so my diet once again consisted of mostly whole plant foods. I cooked and baked from scratch to feed my family delicious, nutritious food as my mother had done all those years ago.

Plant-based eating patterns explained

Plant-based eating is not a new concept, with cultures around the world eating this way for centuries.

Plant-forward and **plant-predominant** diets are terms essentially highlighting that whole or minimally processed plant foods are at the centre of your diet, with animal-derived foods forming a very small part. **Plant-based** is usually used to signify a 100 per cent plant-exclusive diet, mostly whole plant foods.

Being vegan is based on an ethical philosophy of reducing animal exploitation to the best of one's ability. It tells us a vegan doesn't eat any animal products consciously, and avoids all animal-derived products (leather, silk, gelatine etc.) to the best of their ability. While a **vegan diet** means there are no animal products in the diet, it doesn't indicate what the diet is made up of; for example, it could be equally white bread and jam or a diet rich in whole plant foods.

Whole-food, plant-based diet (WFPB)

A WFPB diet is based on eating a variety of minimally processed or whole plant foods, and includes vegetables, fruits, whole grains, legumes, nuts, seeds, and herbs and spices. I would like to include mushrooms, starchy tubers and soya specifically into this way of eating because of their numerous benefits. While people may eat the occasional processed vegan treat, it is a plant-exclusive way of eating.

Eating an anti-inflammatory plant-based or plant-predominant diet encourages a healthy gut microbiome. Optimizing gut health and reducing inflammation are the building blocks for hormonal and overall health.

By eating a variety of whole plant foods, you can get enough calories, all the macronutrients (protein, fat and carbohydrates) in adequate amounts, and in addition, countless phytochemicals, micronutrients and cancer-fighting antioxidants not really found elsewhere in our food. All these foods can be culturally adapted, and there is no need to feel you are missing out.

A note of caution: If you have a history of **disordered eating**, it might not be appropriate for you to rapidly change your current diet, as you may find it triggering. If you do consider moving to a plant-based way of eating, please do so with a qualified professional who can guide you to avoid slipping into restrictive habits.

Components of a whole-food plant-based diet
Fruit

Eat all fruit, especially berries. Fruit has fibre so the sugar in fruit gets absorbed slowly, unlike fruit juices. Eating fruit lowers one's risk of type 2 diabetes, and if one already has diabetes, eating fruit has been shown to lower the risk of complications from type 2 diabetes.

Vegetables

All vegetables, especially green leafy vegetables and cruciferous vegetables (spinach, collard greens, kale, pak choi, broccoli, chard etc.), are packed with fibre and antioxidants.

Legumes

Beans, peas, lentils and pulses are especially rich in fibre and protein. Increased dietary fibre has been shown to predict weight loss in women. Legumes form an essential part of the daily diet of all long-living societies.

Intact whole grains

These could be as close to the original (oat groats, quinoa, wild or black/red rice, millet, spelt, amaranth, barley etc.). Minimally processed grains (e.g. steel-cut or rolled oats, wholewheat pasta, lentil pasta, wholemeal seeded bread, brown rice, brown rice noodles) still have plenty of fibre and micronutrients.

Complex starchy carbohydrates

These include root vegetables or tubers including sweet potatoes, regular potatoes with the skin, yam, tapioca, Jerusalem artichoke etc. They help keep you satiated for longer and are rich in fibre, minerals and vitamins.

Nuts and seeds

These are rich in nutrients such as vitamin E and omega-3 fatty acids (walnuts, flax and chia). Remember to opt for raw over roasted and salted, where possible with fewer harmful advanced glycation end products (**AGEs**) that damage tissues.

Herbs and spices

These are extremely high in antioxidants. Basil, **coriander (cilantro)**, parsley, cumin, turmeric, cinnamon etc. can help to add flavour and boost nutritional value of dishes.

Soya

This deserves a separate mention, even though it is a bean. Soya is considered a high-quality plant protein with all nine essential amino acids arranged in a similar proportion to animal protein, such as egg white, but without its harmful effects. Aim daily for two to four portions of minimally processed soya such as soya milk, tofu, tempeh, miso, natto as they are rich in fibre, protein, healthful fats and vitamins, unless you are allergic (rare, 3–6 in 1000 people). I discuss all the reasons why soya should form a daily part of your diet in perimenopause and menopause in Chapter 14.

Mushrooms

These contain many healthful properties and belong to the fungi group. They are a good source of fibre, contain protein and other micronutrients. Mushrooms when eaten regularly, even in small quantities as part of a diverse diet, may help reduce the risk of breast cancer. They are safest when eaten cooked.

Water

Make water your drink of choice rather than sugar-sweetened drinks, juices, squashes etc. I suggest keeping caffeine-containing drinks to before midday to avoid sleep disruption in women around menopause. Herbal teas are a great way of hydrating. Use sugar, salt and oil minimally (a notable exception is extra virgin olive oil) as flavourings, as benefits of these condiments to menopausal health are minimal.

Foods to crowd out

When you focus on what you're adding into the diet rather than what you're removing, this becomes a joyful process. Think abundance rather than deprivation.

Most ultra-processed foods are usually full of fat, unwanted additives and sugar and are mostly lacking in fibre. These inflammatory foods fuel ill health. These include shop-bought cakes, cookies, pastries, sugar-sweetened beverages and fizzy drinks. Drinking shop-bought fruit juices is not a good idea in general, as these usually have no fibre and are high in **free sugars**. It is always better to stick with the whole fruit.

Limit or exclude most animal-derived foods, especially red meat, processed meats, chicken, cow's milk, cheese and eggs. These products often contain high levels of harmful saturated fat, POPs (persistent organic pollutants are poisonous chemical substances that break down slowly and get into food chains as a result), pesticides, antibiotics etc. and often test positive to pathogenic microorganisms. No animal product contains any fibre, with studies confirming increased inflammation and risk of chronic disease when eaten regularly, as it is in a typical Western diet. Low carbohydrate high animal protein or high animal fat diets are consistently associated with worse outcomes, especially long-term increased death rates. Dairy yoghurt may have a neutral effect on health. Fish is thought to be healthy because of its omega-3 fatty acids, which we can easily get from the same algae source the fish gets it from (Chapter 16). Fish, especially the larger varieties such as tuna, salmon and cod, may have significant levels of hormone disruptors, antibiotics, pesticides and heavy metals such as mercury.

Limiting sugar, salt and oil intake can bring significant health benefits in menopause. I suggest gradually reducing this over time using them as flavourings rather than over consuming. Over a few months, our palates get used to less salt, sugar and oil. Salt stiffens our blood vessels and raises blood pressure (hypertension) when consumed in excess, while free sugars can worsen hot flushes and cause tooth decay. Most oils are a dense source of calories and also release harmful products (AGEs) that speed up ageing when heated to high temperatures. An exception is extra virgin olive oil (Chapter 13).

Getting started

If you are new to eating plant-based, go slow at first so your body and your gut bacteria get used to higher amounts of healthy fibre. It can take as little as three weeks to transition completely to a plant-based diet or as long as three to six months, depending on your starting point. Focus on adding more colour to your plate and practise mindful and intuitive eating.

I like to meet my patients where they are at as it can feel overwhelming if you are not used to this way of eating. My advice is to consider adding as many whole plant foods as you are comfortable with into your daily diet, with a final aim of 10–13 portions of fruit and vegetables daily.

A portion is what fits in the palm of your hand or 80 grams. Berries and a banana for breakfast, a couple of fruits or hummus with vegetable crudités as snacks and a large salad or vegetable soup for lunch or dinner should easily get you to ten portions of fruits and vegetables in a day.

You are in charge

My advice is to focus more on foods to include in your day rather than what you think you must give up. Instead of approaching a food, be it cake or cauliflower, as 'good' or 'bad', saying 'I choose not to' or 'I don't want it' rather than 'I really shouldn't' or 'I can't' allows you to be in control, rather than the food being in control.

I find this mindset is helpful not just for those of you who wish to stop the never-ending cycle of dieting but also for those who wish to manage perimenopause and menopause and chronic lifestyle conditions. I find this approach of being in charge versus denial or restriction works better for most people to help them adopt a healthier attitude and change the fractured relationship many of us have with food.

Inch your way to eating plant-based for better health

While there is no one diet proven to be best for health, all experts agree that whole or minimally processed plant foods promote good health and reduce our risk of chronic disease (heart disease, dementia, type 2 diabetes, certain cancers, obesity), all seen in women in menopause at higher rates.

My advice to you is to make small sustainable changes and inch your way towards a scientifically proven whole-food, plant-based way of eating and good health. This fibre-rich diet prevents surges of insulin and blood sugar, making weight gain, diabetes and vasomotor symptoms of menopause easier to manage. A plant-based diet has been shown to be beneficial for all aspects of women's health, whether it is painful periods, PCOS, endometriosis or recovering from surgery.

The evidence for eating plants for perimenopause and menopause

Studies evaluating diet quality or dietary patterns have shown an association between lower intensity of psychological and physical symptoms, sleep disorders, and vasomotor (hot flushes, night sweats), urogenital (bladder) symptoms in those who have a higher consumption of vegetables, whole grains and unprocessed foods.[1,2,3] Also, an increased intensity of these menopausal symptoms is associated with ultra-processed foods, saturated fat and sugars. There appears to be an association between both high caffeine intake and type of fat intake (saturated fat worsens) with the intensity of menopausal symptoms experienced.[4] Larger studies of better quality would be helpful to clarify details of dietary intake, but are not yet available.

A trial showed women who followed a plant-based diet with the addition of half a cup of mature soybeans daily reduced their severe and moderate hot flush symptoms by an incredible 84 per cent, as I discuss in some more detail in Chapter 14.[5]

Vegans were found to have less bothersome menopausal symptoms compared to their counterparts.[6] Women who snacked on fresh fruit and vegetables had fewer vasomotor symptoms than those who snacked on sugary and fatty snack foods, butter etc.[7]

Current evidence suggests that low-fat, plant-based diets are associated with beneficial effects on body composition and weight, but further studies are needed to confirm these results in post-menopausal women.[8]

The Mediterranean diet pattern (a diet full of plant foods with olive oil, some fish and poultry and little dairy) along with other healthy habits may help the primary prevention of bone, metabolic and cardiovascular diseases in the post-menopausal period. The consumption of healthy plant foods that have anti-inflammatory and antioxidant properties is associated with a small but significant decrease in blood pressure, reduction of fat mass and improvement in cholesterol levels.[8,9,10,11,12]

Interestingly, diet may influence the age of natural menopause by around 18 months. A large UK-based study of more than 35,000 women aged 35–69 years found that there was an association between higher intakes of oily fish and fresh legumes and a delay of the natural menopause, while higher GI refined foods such as white pasta and rice on the other hand were associated with an earlier menopause.[4,13]

Find your why

Some of the reasons my patients say they want to change to a plant-based way of eating include:

- 'I want to feel healthy.'
- 'I want to feel energetic.'

- 'I want to recover faster from exercise.'
- 'I don't want to feel hungry or tired all the time.'
- 'I want to stop counting calories.'
- 'I want to reduce my medications if possible.'
- 'I want to be around for my grandkids.'

My own reasons for eating a plant-exclusive diet include my earlier menopause, for improving my general health, for combating climate change and because I am vegan. I want to remain healthy to continue to enjoy life with my family and loved ones, while continuing to help people.

Menopause mantra: *Food for thought*

A whole-food, plant-based (WFPB) diet is beneficial in menopause as it:

- reduces inflammation and oxidative stress
- improves insulin resistance
- promotes weight loss and weight maintenance
- lowers excess oestrogen levels
- promotes healthy gut bacteria.

To move towards a WFPB diet:

- focus on fruits, vegetables, legumes, whole grains, nuts and seeds
- make water your drink of choice
- limit animal foods
- avoid or minimize ultra-processed foods
- remember that low carbohydrate high animal protein or high animal fat diets are consistently associated with worse outcomes, especially long-term increased death rates.

12

Menopause bloating: Gut health in menopause

Case: Susan sat in front of me concerned that her bloating had got worse over the last 12 months. She had suffered from constipation for years. Nothing had changed in her diet. She had been having a few panic attacks and was not sleeping very well. She was in her early 50s and still getting her periods, although not as regularly.

Before I could conclude that Susan's bloating was menopause related, I took a detailed medical history, including any changes in appetite, loss of weight, past medical and gynaecological issues, her bowel habits, family history of cancers, including bowel and ovarian cancers, and performed a thorough examination. In these situations, an abdominal and pelvic ultrasound scan is reasonable along with some blood tests. They were all normal in her particular case, but sometimes there can be serious underlying conditions.

Susan's dietary habits had not changed, but she was eating a standard Western diet that was deficient in fibre. She felt the onset of menopause had made her existing symptoms of bloating and constipation worse.

Fibre

Like most people in the UK, Susan's diet did not have enough fibre. Only one in ten people meet the recommended target of 30 g/day, with the average intake being a meagre 17 g/day for women.[1,2] Humans have evolved eating a diverse range of plants that regularly contributed to around 100 g of fibre per day over millions of years.[3] Eating whole plants allows you to hit your target for fibre rather easily as only plant foods have fibre. There is minimal fibre in ultra-processed foods and none in animal foods.

One result of this is that constipation is a real problem for many in the UK as most eat a standard diet made up of close to 60 per cent highly processed foods, significantly increasing the risk of heart disease, strokes and high blood pressure.[4] Susan admitted to me that the laxatives seemed to have stopped working, as they often do.

As Dr Denis Burkitt, a British doctor who worked for years in Africa, famously observed, 'Societies that eat unrefined foods produce large stools and build small hospitals; societies that eat fibre-depleted foods produce small stools and build large hospitals.' Constipation, diverticulitis and bowel cancer risks are significantly increased when diets lack fibre.[5]

Prebiotics, probiotics and post-biotics

We have about 100 trillion bacteria living inside our gut, both good and bad, along with other microorganisms (fungi, archaea, viruses etc.). Beneficial gut bacteria (also found in food and certain supplements), known as **probiotics**, feast on **prebiotics** or feeding material found in fibre-rich plant foods, producing healthy by-products called **post-biotics** such as short chain fatty acids (SCFA) that are critical not just to our general health (gut, heart, brain health) but also to our hormonal health. These good bacteria keep the bad bugs such as *E. coli* and *Salmonella* and thrush-causing *Candida* in check, all of which can negatively impact women's health.

The significant lack of fibre in a typical Western diet means that the healthy colonies of bacteria such as *Firmicutes* do not flourish. Instead, the gut harbours an environment that allows inflammatory colonies of microbes such as *Bacteroides*, *Bilophila wadsworthia*, *Clostridium* and enteroinvasive *E. coli* to take root, releasing endotoxins such as amines, sulphides and secondary bile salts amongst other harmful substances that damage the delicate gut lining over time and promote ill health.

The American Gut Project, the largest study to date of the gut microbiome, found that people who ate 30 different plant foods each week had a more diverse gut microbiome, and produced more of the beneficial short-chain fatty acids, compared with those who ate ten or fewer plant foods. This number is rather easy to achieve on a whole-food plant-based diet packed with fibre, the food that the good gut bacteria thrive on, and is highly unlikely to be reached on a standard Western diet, even if one takes fibre supplements. It is easy to improve one's gut microbiome in a matter of days and weeks with a healthy plant-based diet.[6]

The oestrobolome

There is evidence to suggest our oral, vaginal and gut microbiome are regulated and altered by oestrogen levels.

There is a collection of microbes in our gut, part of the gut microbiome, known as the oestrobolome, which is one of the principal regulators and recyclers of circulating oestrogens (and testosterone and progesterone) in our body. The oestrobolome can break down excess oestrogen that the body is trying to get rid of, which it does by binding unwanted oestrogen to the fibre derived from the plants we eat, excreting it out in our faeces.

This trapping of oestrogen by the fibre in the food we eat prevents the excess hormones from re-entering the blood circulation via the liver, by a mechanism called the enterohepatic circulation. Those on plant-based diets tend to excrete two to three times more of the unwanted oestrogen. This is important information that can further encourage us to include more plants in our diet, as we know many women's health conditions, such as PCOS, endometriosis, fibroids, adenomyosis and certain cancers such as breast and womb cancers, are associated with higher levels of excess oestrogen, produced from excess body fat and also found in the animal foods we eat.

Eating a fibre-rich plant-predominant diet can help promote a healthy oestrobolome.

Gut health in menopause

Symptoms of functional gastrointestinal disorders including fullness, bloating, abdominal pain and altered gastrointestinal (GI) motility appear to be more common in perimenopause and menopause. Whether dropping levels of oestrogen and progesterone are responsible for this or the rather complex relation between our gut–brain axis is hard to confirm, as large studies are lacking. A combination of both factors is likely to be responsible for some of the changes seen in gut health around menopause.

As levels of oestrogen and progesterone drop, research suggests that menopause is associated with a lower gut microbiome diversity, with a trend for the microbiome to become more similar to that of men. Gut microbiome diversity appears to plateau around age 40. There also appears to be an increased permeability of the gut barrier, allowing microbes to cross into the cells.[7] Reduced gut microbial diversity appears to increase the risk of obesity, cardiovascular disease, metabolic syndrome and other chronic illnesses, which are seen at higher rates in menopause.[8,9] These observations are from small studies, as currently there is a lack of large reliable studies on gut health in perimenopause and menopause.

Gut–brain axis

There is a bidirectional communication network that links our gut to the brain, allowing the brain to influence intestinal activities and vice versa. Mood and cognitive changes, anxiety and depression seen more commonly in perimenopause and menopause can therefore be associated with GI disruptions such as constipation, diarrhoea, reflux, abdominal pain and bloating,[10] and similarly a less diverse gut microbiome seen in menopause and in conditions like **irritable bowel syndrome (IBS)** may increase psychological comorbidities.[11]

Serotonin, a neurotransmitter best known in the regulation of mood (feel-good hormone) and gut motility, is influenced by the gut microbiome through complex mechanisms. Low levels of serotonin in the brain may cause anxiety, depression and problems with sleep.[12,13]

In simple words, a healthy gut microbiome may help improve mood in menopause.

Helping yourself

All six lifestyle pillars can help you improve your gut health via the gut microbiome. Managing stress and improving mood through sleep, positive social connections and exercise while avoiding alcohol and tobacco as well as inappropriate use of antibiotics can all help improve gut and general health. Adopting a diverse, fibre-rich, plant-predominant diet is a great way to improve microbial diversity in your gut.

Bloating on a plant-based diet

Many women are worried about this. Over time, most people find that they are less, or not at all, bloated on a plant-based diet, as the gut microbiome changes to healthy colonies of bacteria that know how to deal with fibre. Nutritionist Rohini shares her top tips to beat bloating on a plant-based diet.

Rohini's tips to avoid bloating on a plant-based diet

- Introduce beans and lentils gradually. Start with smaller lentils first.
- Rinse canned beans and lentils.
- Soak dried beans for 6–10 hours before rinsing and cooking.
- Cook beans and lentils until soft (be able to mash with fork).
- Be mindful when eating and chew each mouthful slowly.
- Enjoy herbs and spices such as peppermint, asafoetida and ginger.
- Drink enough water as you increase the fibre in your diet.

Menopause mantra: *Only plants have fibre*

- Dropping levels of oestrogen can make the gut microbiome less diverse in menopause.
- Symptoms of bloating, fullness, reflux and slowing of gut motility are common in menopause.
- A link between the gut and the brain (gut–brain axis) may influence menopause symptoms.
- Improving mood and lowering stress in menopause can help with bowel symptoms.
- Only plants have fibre and adopting a plant-predominant diet promotes a healthy gut microbiome.
- Addressing other lifestyle factors such as exercise and sleep may also help improve gut health.
- Seek urgent medical advice for persistent bowel issues, or if there is rectal bleeding.

13

Cravings: Benefits of limiting sugar, salt and oil in menopause

'Every time I eat sugar or sugary foods, my hot flushes seem to get worse. Is that possible?' asked Maria, a patient of mine in her late 40s.

In this section, I discuss the benefits of reducing salt, sugar and oil for women in perimenopause and menopause. There are many misconceptions about various forms of sugar and the types of salt and oil, that I intend to clarify.

Salt, oil and sugar are often viewed as essential for tasty palatable food, but you will find the recipes in Part 4, 'Menopause Morsels', are packed with flavour with minimal use of these ingredients. The flavour comes from the use of herbs, spices, aromatics such as cinnamon, cumin, garlic and ginger which pack a punch and have numerous health benefits.

This is not to demonize salt, oil or sugar, which are generally fine in small amounts, but rather to provide suggestions for prioritizing nutrient-dense foods, which is especially important for women as we get older. It's also a question of adapting your palate with small changes over time. In general, use sugar, salt and oil as flavourings rather than in excess.

A note of caution: If you have a history of disordered eating, it might not be appropriate for you to focus on reducing or eliminating sugar, salt or oil. It is more important to prioritize your wellbeing over restriction.

Sugar intake in menopause

The years around menopause are characterized by fluctuations of our sex hormones which in turn have an impact on a reduction in lean body mass and an increase in fat deposition, increasing the risk of developing insulin resistance (IR) as we get older. Along with insulin and cortisol, our sex hormones influence glucose regulation and affect hormones like leptin and ghrelin (hunger hormones).

Insulin resistance occurs when our cells and tissues become resistant over time to the action of insulin, a hormone produced by the pancreas, the role of which is to shift the glucose broken down from the food we eat from our bloodstream into our cells to provide energy. This results in rising blood sugar levels. Insulin resistance is seen in women with PCOS and also in women carrying excess weight, increasing the risk of type 2 diabetes, heart disease, obesity and possibly worsening of menopausal vasomotor symptoms (hot flushes and night sweats).

There is evidence to suggest that the hot flushes are less frequent after eating a meal, while hot flushes are experienced more when blood glucose falls between meals.[1] When we eat highly refined sugary foods like cakes and cookies, after an initial rise, there is often a significant drop in blood sugar levels which may be the reason for Maria's observation of more hot flushes after a sugary snack.

Normally, eating a meal with a high glycaemic index (GI), such as white bread with jam, or sugary breakfast cereal, elicits a surge of insulin, as a response to the rapidly rising blood glucose levels. The insulin in turn rapidly lowers blood glucose.

Around menopause, this metabolic flexibility, meaning the ability to switch from fat utilization during fasting to carbohydrate utilization during hyperinsulinemia (raised insulin levels), appears to be reduced as oestrogen levels fall, increasing hunger and cravings.[2]

It is often portrayed in the media that all ill health is down to excess sugar in our diet, but this is not necessarily true.[3] It is important to understand that it is the overall dietary pattern that is important, and not that occasional slice of birthday cake or the holiday indulgence. That said, the amount of sugar we are currently eating as a population is excessive and can contribute to weight gain and its associated health issues.

Added sugars are not necessary in a healthy dietary pattern. Free sugars (which means sugars added to food or drinks, and sugars found naturally in honey, syrups, maple syrup, agave, and sweetened fruit and vegetable juices and smoothies) should not make up more than 5 per cent of the calories you get from food and drink each day. Adults should have no more than 30 g of free sugars a day (roughly equivalent to seven sugar cubes).[4] Artificial sweeteners have not been found to make a significant difference to weight when replacing free sugars and do not have any health benefits.

Sugar is also found in surprisingly high quantities in certain savoury foods such as pizza, table sauces, low-fat yoghurts, ready meals and most breakfast cereals, so being aware of this will help you limit your added sugar intake and extra calories.

Dental health in menopause

You may be surprised to know oestrogen receptors are found in the mouth (oral mucosa) and salivary glands. As oestrogen levels drop around menopause, this can lead to oral discomfort, increasing gum disease, dry or burning mouth.[5]

As a society, tooth decay is closely related to our intake of free sugars found in hyper-palatable foods such as candy, cakes, breakfast cereals, squashes and juices. Reducing these in general, and if you do eat them, limiting them to mealtimes, rinsing out your mouth after eating is important. Paying attention to your oral hygiene (brushing and flossing daily) with regular visits to the dentist can help limit tooth decay in menopause.

'But fruit has sugar'

You should not limit the amount of fruit you eat in menopause. The idea that fruit should be limited as it has too much sugar is false.

I hear this all the time from many of my patients who are frightened to eat most fruit. Women are often falsely concerned about eating any fruit because of the sugar content. I spend a significant amount of time in my clinic encouraging women to eat fruit and not be afraid of the sugar content.

Fruit is one of the healthiest foods that everyone can and should eat plenty of. This common misconception that fruit equals sugar shows the danger of reducing foods to their specific nutrients rather than looking at the whole package. Whole fruits come packaged with beneficial phytonutrients, fibre, vitamins, minerals and water and have consistently been shown to reduce the risk of type 2 diabetes, even at high fruit intakes. Even fruit such as bananas and mangos are in the medium glycaemic index range and are rich in fibre.

The fibre present in all fruit helps slow the absorption of sugar in the bloodstream, which is why fruit juices which contain minimal fibre should be limited or avoided in your daily diet. Although it's a great source of fibre, dried fruit should be limited to a serving or a small handful a day if you are concerned about your weight, as it's a concentrated source of energy in a small package.

For maximum health benefits in menopause, aim to eat a variety of fruit daily as part of a diverse diet. All whole fresh or frozen fruit is health-promoting in menopause and of all fruits, berries pack the greatest antioxidant punch.

A note of caution: Avoid restrictive diets such as a fruit-only or a completely raw diet, as it is difficult to meet all nutritional requirements essential for health, especially in the long-term.

Salt intake in menopause

Common salt is sodium chloride. Sodium is a mineral playing an essential role in our body, helping transport water around the body and in transmitting messages between our brain and the rest of our body. The kidneys regulate the amount of sodium in the body. If the kidneys can't remove enough sodium, it builds up in the blood which can cause problems over time.

Sodium sensitivity increases in perimenopause with women noticing changes because of fluid retention, with swelling or oedema of legs and hands, puffy face and baggy eyelids, often on waking.[6]

Dietary salt intake is a known risk factor for hypertension or high blood pressure, which stiffens our blood vessels and increases our incidence of heart attacks, stroke, kidney disease and vascular dementia as we get older.

The average person in the UK consumes about 8 g of salt every day, while in the USA and India, it is about 9 g per day, with China at almost 11 g of salt per day, considerably higher than the WHO advice which is for adults to consume no more than 5 g of salt (2000 mg of sodium) on a daily basis.[7] According to the British Dietetic Association, around three-quarters of the salt we eat is added to the food we buy.

Table or cooking salt is sodium chloride, as is Himalayan salt, pink salt, rock salt or sea salt, so please do not get misled into believing these alternatives are in any way healthier for you. They tend to be more expensive than regular salt and are also not iodized, with no robust evidence or studies to show they are better for us. It is best to limit our salt intake.

A reduction in dietary sodium not only decreases blood pressure and the incidence of hypertension but is also associated with a reduction in death and disability from cardiovascular diseases.[8]

Ways to reduce salt intake

Skipping or limiting high-sodium foods such as crisps, stock cubes, cheese and processed meat can help reduce salt in the diet. It is a good idea to read the label as foods that are marketed as healthy such as certain pasta sauces and breakfast cereals are often high in sugar and salt.

The DASH diet (Dietary Approaches to Stop Hypertension) or a whole-food, plant-based diet are both excellent dietary choices to help you reduce your salt intake. Simply eating more whole plant foods is a great way to reduce your daily salt intake.

Potassium chloride as a substitute for common salt has been shown to help in reducing blood pressure in some studies. Experts say more robust studies are needed before recommending population-wide replacement of sodium chloride with potassium-enriched salt substitutes.

Use fresh and dried herbs, spices, citrus, vinegars, pepper and mustard as seasoning so you need to add less salt. This is how we have designed our recipes in *Finding Me in Menopause* to make them so delicious. If desired, I recommend adding salt at the table using a salt mill to get the taste.

Oil intake in menopause

Oils are a dense source of calories, with one tablespoon of oil containing around 120 calories. Given that the incidence of medically defined obesity and overweight is over 60 per cent for women, calorie restriction in some form is necessary for many of us. Eating healthy whole fats which come with fibre unlike their extracted oils is generally preferable, especially if you are planning to lose weight healthily in menopause.

Chemically speaking, free oils are chains of carbon found in a purified state. The extraction process removes most of the other ingredients of the whole food. As a result, most oils do not have the abundance of phytonutrients, vitamins and minerals that occur naturally in whole plant foods such as nuts and seeds.

Cooking with oils heated to high temperatures releases advanced glycation end products (AGEs) – glycoproteins that cause tissue damage, ageing, arterial stiffness, **oxidative stress** and hormonal disruption. For cooking at higher temperatures, rapeseed or avocado oil are good options due to their higher smoking points, but should still be kept to a minimum.

Small amounts of oil can be added if you wish, especially if it improves your enjoyment of food. However, for most people there is no evidence to suggest that oils have to be an essential part of our diets.

High-quality cold-pressed extra virgin olive oil (**EVOO**) used raw or in low-temperature cooking can be useful if you have a small appetite, you are finding it hard to maintain weight or for those who would like to gain weight. You might also simply enjoy the taste. Hemp seed oil, flax oil or walnut oil are some other omega 3-rich options.

Olive oil in menopause

Olive oil is a good source of unsaturated fats and **polyphenols**, which can help reduce inflammation, metabolic syndrome, maintain healthy blood sugar and blood pressure levels and promote weight loss as part of a Mediterranean-style diet (fruits, vegetables, beans and healthy fats), based on observational and experimental studies.[9]

EVOO and canola (also known as rapeseed) oil both contain monounsaturated fats and polyunsaturated fats (MUFA, PUFA), with studies showing benefit for the brain and the heart, especially as we get older. These oils in particular are always preferable to eating butter (mostly saturated fat), ghee, coconut oil or eating trans fats found in ultra-processed foods, all of which may slow blood flow for hours after a fatty meal. Tropical oils such as coconut oil should also be avoided as they raise LDL cholesterol levels consistently, like animal-derived fats, and are implicated in causing heart disease.

Choosing healthy fats

There is a distinction between oil and healthy fats, the latter of which are essential for everyone, especially children, pregnant women and older adults. Fat can help with the absorption of certain nutrients, such as fat-soluble vitamins A, D, E and K. A range of delicious nuts, seeds and avocados provides healthy fats, without needing to reach for the oil.

Authentic EVOO can certainly be a useful addition of healthy fats to one's diet in menopause, but it tends to be expensive and hard to come by, so it is worth checking the credentials of the company you are buying the oil from.

Oil-free cooking

If you wish to reduce the amount of oil when cooking, and as a result the number of calories in a dish, there is a healthy way to do this. Start by gradually reducing the oil you use to cook with by half every week until you are using little or none. Alongside this, you can learn to cook, sauté, roast with hot water, vinegar, stock or wine, all of which can be great substitutions depending on the meal. I use many of these techniques when I cook and in the flavoursome recipes in this book. You will be surprised how good your dishes can taste with little or no oil.

As a South Indian growing up in Kolkata, both coconut oil and mustard oil evoke happy memories. If you want the flavour of oil in certain dishes as I do sometimes, consider adding a small amount of cold-pressed oil to a dish, for example, EVOO to a salad, a few drops of mustard oil to Bengali dishes, a few drops of warm coconut oil to South Indian vegetable dishes or sesame oil to Chinese dishes.

Menopause mantra: *There are many delicious and natural ways to reduce my salt, sugar and oil intake*

- Use salt, oil and sugar (SOS) as flavourings rather than in excess.
- Use herbs, spices like cinnamon, flavoured vinegars and lemon juice as alternatives.
- Eat a variety of colourful fibre-rich whole fruits without concern about sugar content.
- Limit fizzy sugar-sweetened beverages, fruit juices and free sugars to reduce menopausal symptoms and improve heart and dental health.
- Replace sugar and sweeteners with mashed banana, applesauce, dates or fresh or dried fruit when you can in cooking and baking.
- If you choose an oil, choose cold-pressed extra virgin olive oil over most other oils.
- Sauté using hot water or stock instead.
- Eating healthy fats from nuts, seeds, tofu, avocados and EVOO promotes good health.

14

Soy good: The benefits of adding soya to your diet

Soya is good, soya is safe, soya is healthy, based on current scientific evidence. You may have read otherwise. Unaware of the science that strongly supports the consumption of soya as a healthful addition to everyone's diet at all ages and stages of life, many people who would benefit, including women in perimenopause and menopause, avoid it completely when there is absolutely no need to.

There is a mistaken belief that soya is a hormonal disruptor when in reality, it is quite the opposite. For a humble bean, soya has so much unnecessary controversy surrounding it, despite being consumed safely by healthy populations all around the world for thousands of years to their benefit.

My aim in this chapter is to dispel myths, and using scientific research and studies, explain why it is a good idea to include soya in your daily diet.

All about soya

Soya (or 'soy' as it is known in North America) has a positive role in managing perimenopause and menopause for several reasons. In fact, all legumes (beans, lentils, peas) are great for perimenopause and menopause, and should be part of all diets as they promote health, but the soyabean deserves a special mention. The soyabean is technically classified as a legume and has been consumed in China for at least 3000 years.

Soya is a high-quality plant protein source

All plants contain all nine essential amino acids, building blocks that our body cannot make and which must come from external sources. What makes soya remarkable is that it contains all the nine essential amino acids in a similar proportion to animal protein (in fact to egg white, often promoted as the best protein source), making it a high-quality protein source but without any of the undesirable effects of animal foods. The majority of soya products have high protein quality scores.[1,2] Soya is also very low in undesirable saturated fats found in high amounts in many animal products. It is a rich source of fibre to feed our gut microbiome, healthy polyunsaturated fats (PUFAs), resistant starch and a good source of vitamins and minerals such as calcium, iron, potassium, folate and magnesium.

'Soya will mess up my hormones'

When I ask my patients to eat soya, they usually say they have heard soya can mess with their hormones and ask if this is true. The short and long answer to that is a categoric 'no'. With hundreds of scientific studies resulting from over 30 years of rigorous research on soya and more than 2000 soya-related peer-reviewed articles published, the message is clear: soya is a healthy addition to any dietary pattern. Unless one is allergic, eating soya is healthful for every age and for all genders. Soya plays an especially beneficial role in reproductive and menopausal health. Consuming soya appears to counteract hormone disruption.[3,4]

Plant oestrogens are safe

A great deal of misconceptions stem from the fact that soya contains phytoestrogens (plant oestrogens) which resemble the oestrogen hormone found in our body but with much weaker oestrogen activity. These plant compounds occur in nature in other plant foods but are found in higher quantities in soya.

Isoflavones found in soya beans, chickpeas, beans, fruits and pistachio nuts, lignans found in flaxseeds, sesame seeds and whole-grain cereals, and coumestans found in split peas, pinto beans, lima beans and alfalfa sprouts are three of the best-known group of phytoestrogens. Daidzein and genistein are the two main types of isoflavones in soya beans.

The difference between plant oestrogens and mammalian oestrogen

Soya binds preferentially to the beta oestrogen receptors in our cells while the mammalian oestrogen found in our own body fat and in animal-derived foods binds to both the alpha and beta oestrogen receptors. This selective mechanism allows soya isoflavones to cleverly mimic oestrogen in some tissues of the body while in others it has an oestrogen-blocking effect, for example, promoting bone health but reducing breast and uterine cancer risks. This dual action, known as a selective estrogen receptor modulator (SERM) effect, is responsible for many of the positive health effects of soya that are separate from its other properties of being rich in fibre and protein. Isn't nature remarkable?

Soya for vasomotor symptoms of menopause

There are several studies of variable quality to show that regular consumption of soya can help relieve hot flushes in menopause.[5,6] Some of these studies have looked at populations that consume soya regularly as part of their diet while others have studied women on isoflavone supplements for a period of time.[5,6,7,29,30]

A promising study using soya as food instead of supplements is the Women's Study for the Alleviation of Vasomotor Symptoms (WAVS) published in 2021. Dr Neal Barnard and his team used a combination of a low-fat, plant-based diet and just half a cup of cooked whole soybeans or 86 g (containing around 55–60 g of isoflavones) daily for a period of 12 weeks and found it was associated with reduced frequency and severity of hot flushes and improved quality of life in vasomotor, psychosocial, physical, and sexual symptoms in post-menopausal women in the USA. In fact, the majority of women in the group on this diet became free of moderate-to-severe hot flushes (84 per cent). That is powerful information to show how what we eat can make a significant difference to quality of life, and especially important for those who cannot take HRT for their vasomotor symptoms.[8]

The average daily consumption of isoflavones in a typical Western diet is a dismal 1–2 mg of isoflavones compared to 15–60 mg/day in Asian countries, where there is typically a high consumption of soya and its derived foodstuffs.[9]

Soya helps build bone, promotes heart health, helps with weight management and reduces cancer risk. There are many other health benefits of including soya bean products in your diet in perimenopause and menopause. Soya, when consumed regularly, may help promote bone health and reduce the risk of osteoporosis.[9,10,11]

Soya beans contain several constituents able to modulate the development of cancer at several levels, namely initiation, promotion and cancer progression.[12,13]

Soya and cancer risk

Higher intake of soy and soy isoflavones is found to be inversely associated with risk of cancer incidence. The beneficial role of soya against cancer might be primarily attributed to the soya isoflavones.[12]

An analysis of 14 studies published in the *American Journal of Clinical Nutrition* showed that increased intake of soya resulted in a 26 per cent reduction in prostate cancer risk. On the other hand, studies have shown consumption of dairy, even at relatively low doses, to be associated with a 25 per cent increased risk of aggressive prostate cancer.[12,13,14,15,16]

Soya reduces breast cancer risk

When started early in childhood or young adult life, consuming as little as one portion of soya daily may reduce breast cancer risks.

The Shanghai Women's Health Study over seven years consisting of thousands of women observed over seven years has been the largest and most detailed study of soya and breast cancer risk in a population that has a high soya consumption. Women who ate the most soya had a 59 per cent lower risk of pre-menopausal breast cancer, compared with those who ate the lowest amounts of soya. A follow-up analysis of the same women over 13 years found further impressive results, with a 22 per cent lower risk of breast cancer when comparing the highest to lowest intakes of soya during adulthood.[17,18,19]

Even among women with breast cancer, soya consumption is found to be significantly associated with decreased risk of death and recurrence.[20,21]

Soya lowers the risk of several lifestyle-related cancers

The risk of certain gynaecological cancers such as womb (endometrial)[3,13] and ovarian cancer as well as other cancers such as bowel and liver cancers is also lower in those who consume soya regularly. This anti-cancer property is partly due to one of the isoflavones found in soya called genistein, which is found to inhibit angiogenesis or new blood vessel formation, an important step in the development of cancer.[22]

Gut health

Soya is good for the bowel, including for those with inflammatory bowel conditions such as ulcerative colitis.

Soya is cardioprotective

There are heart benefits too from soya, with fermented versions of soya such as tempeh being particularly cardio-protective. When consumed regularly, soya has been consistently shown to help and improve many of the metabolic markers, such as glucose control, biomarkers of inflammation and oxidative stress, and cholesterol and triglyceride levels.

Replacing red meat with plant proteins including soya foods, beans, and nuts was associated with a 14 per cent lower risk of heart disease in a large study,[23, 24] while another very large study of half a million adults found those who ate soya for more than four days a week had a 25 per cent lower risk of death from heart attack.[25] Twice as many women die from heart disease as men, especially in menopause, so all the more reason to eat soya regularly.

Soya and cognition in menopause

The soya isoflavone, daidzein, may play a role in women in post-menopause in helping prevent age-related memory loss and reduce cognitive decline.[26] Larger studies are needed, as those available currently are inconclusive when it comes to the effect of soya on the brain. In the meantime, continue to enjoy soya for its numerous other benefits.

Soya does not affect fertility

Despite the misconceptions, reproductive health is not adversely affected by soya in men or women and may help improve fertility levels. Asian countries have historically consumed soya as part of healthful dietary patterns for thousands of years, without an adverse impact on male or female fertility. Consuming soya or soya-based formulas from infancy also has no negative effects on general or reproductive health.

Human studies consistently show that eating soya foods does not raise oestrogen levels, disrupt hormonal balance, or reduce testosterone concentrations in men.[3,4]

Soya and thyroid issues

Coexistent thyroid dysfunction is not a contraindication to consume soya in the amounts we have recommended above. Soya has no significant effect on the thyroid hormones.[3,27] *However, check with your doctor if you are in any doubt.* The general recommendation is to consume your thyroid medication (usually levothyroxine) at least 30–60 minutes before breakfast, as soya and thyroxine compete for the same receptors in the thyroid.

You should also ensure adequate iodine intake, with a supplement if needed (150 mcg) as most standard Western diets are deficient in iodine, especially in places such as the UK where salt is not iodized.

You can be an equol producer too

It appears that consuming soya from childhood or adolescence allows higher levels of protective equol to be produced by our gut microbiome by breaking down the isoflavone daidzein found in soya. Plant-predominant diets, especially those containing good quantities of soya, encourage the production of equol which is believed to block the potentially negative effects of excess human oestrogen and to be one of the reasons behind soya's cancer prevention benefits.

Recommended servings of soya in menopause

Whatever your diet, you should aim to consume two to four portions of whole or minimally processed soya foods daily, depending on your level of activity. One portion is a 200 ml cup of soya milk or soya yoghurt or 80 g, which is roughly a handful of tofu, tempeh, edamame beans, natto or mature soya beans. I suggest rotating the types of soya bean products, so you get to eat a variety throughout the week, along with other colourful plant foods. Some people with higher calorie needs, such as athletes and those approaching menopause, can benefit from eating up to four portions of soya a day. My own diet has included 3–4 portions of soya most days for years.

Two servings of these traditional soya foods per day provide around 15–20 g high quality protein and approximately 20–50 mg of protective isoflavones, with the protein in the soya representing around 20–25 per cent of your total dietary protein intake.

Processed forms of soya

I am often asked about the type of soya one should consume. It is preferable to include whole or minimally processed soya products daily rather than highly processed soya products. It is fine to enjoy the occasional soya sausage or soya-based plant-based meat alternative, especially as you get older, as they are a good protein source. It is also a useful addition for those transitioning to a plant-based way of eating, but they can contain higher levels of salt, sugar and saturated fat, although far less than a traditional pork sausage. In general, however, I encourage you to enjoy the less processed soya most of the time.

Soya protein isolates such as protein powders can be a useful addition for women in the menopause to achieve their protein targets by adding it to a smoothie. My advice remains to always focus more on soya foods that contain fibre, micronutrients, isoflavones as well as the plant protein such a tofu and tempeh. We do know animal whey protein promotes **insulin-like growth factor IGF1**, which in excess levels may worsen diabetes and promote the growth of certain cancers. Reassuringly, high intake of soy protein is not associated with increased cancer risk, unlike high intakes of animal protein.

Fortified vs organic soya products

In the UK, I would recommend choosing fortified soya products even if not labelled organic, such as calcium-set tofu and calcium-fortified soya milk, as these are good sources of essential nutrients. Calcium from soya is just as well absorbed as in dairy products, with soya milk having the added advantage of being vitamin D enriched, which is not the case for cow's milk in the UK. Calcium-set tofu contains approximately 400 mg of calcium per 100 g. A 100 g serving would provide half the recommended daily amount of calcium per day for adults and also contains magnesium, another useful nutrient for healthy bones.

In the UK, almost all the soya used for tofu, tempeh, soya milk and edamame beans (Cauldron tofu, Alpro soya milk, etc.) comes from Asia and Europe, and is certified GMO free.[28]

GM or genetically modified crops have been around since the mid-1990s, with genes added to many commonly consumed crops to make them more resistant to pests, reduce pesticide use, improve nutrient quality, reduce spoilage, and make farming easier. Scientists agree that currently available food derived from GM crops adds no greater risk to human health than non-GM food, but some people remain nervous. If you are worried about consuming GM soya products and live in the USA, Australia or any another country, do check the labels to see if the product is certified GMO free and organic.

Soya allergy

Compared with milk, egg, peanut, and fish allergy, soya allergy is less common. Only a tiny proportion of adults are allergic to soya, no more than 0.3–0.6 per cent of the population, compared to 2–3 per cent who are allergic to dairy. If allergies are suspected it is important to see your doctor as some food allergies can be serious.

Plant-based diets without soya

You can still thrive on a plant-based diet, rich in other beans and lentils, even if you cannot have soya. However, do not deny yourself the benefits of this wonderful bean, unless you are allergic to it. If you have gut health issues or an intolerance or sensitivity to beans rather than a true allergy, consider reintroducing it slowly over time, ideally with the help of a qualified nutrition professional.

Soya and the environment

Originally from Southeast Asia, the soya plant is a nitrogen-fixing legume. The demand for soya is not being driven by those eating plant-based diets. Only around 7 per cent of the soya produced is used for human consumption in foods such as tofu and tempeh. This non-genetically modified soya is still mostly produced in Asia as well as in the USA and Europe. *The answer is not to stop eating soya but to significantly reduce our consumption of animal products.*

Animal agriculture is responsible for 80–85 per cent of soya production globally. Soya cultivation, primarily used for animal feed and some biofuels, is a major driver of deforestation in the Amazon basin. Chicken and eggs have the heaviest soya footprint, followed by pork and farmed salmon.

Much of the controversy arises as a result of soya monocrops grown primarily in the United States, Brazil, and Argentina, with people not realizing how much soya is being grown to fatten animals. The United Nations estimates a need for new land almost twice the size of Switzerland by 2028 in order to grow soya for animal feed.[31]

The Worldwide Fund for Nature (WWF) released data that each human on average consumes 61 kg of soya per year, which is more than 1 kg a week. Most of this soya is being consumed indirectly by us, as it is fed to animals. The production of one litre of cow's milk requires more than 22 times more water and 12 times more land than one litre of soya milk, while generating three times more greenhouse gas emissions.[32,33]

Don't deny yourself the benefits of soya

Soya is particularly beneficial in the years leading up to and during menopause for a number of reasons. Soya can help with weight loss, which helps reduce severity of hot flushes; it is a great source of plant protein, which is often neglected as one gets older. Soya is rich in plant oestrogens that can help reduce hot flushes. Soya also reduces the risk of many common chronic conditions such as heart disease and certain lifestyle-related cancers.

Having seen the scientific data, I hope you feel confident about adding this versatile bean to your diet on a daily basis, if you are not already doing so. I am sure you will enjoy some of my favourite soya-based recipes in Part 4, 'Menopause Morsels'.

Menopause mantra: *Soya is good for me*

- Soya is safe for all ages as part of a varied diet, unless you are allergic.
- Soya is a bean, rich in high quality protein, fibre and micronutrients.
- Soya contains healthy plant oestrogens called isoflavones.
- Soya can reduce hot flushes in menopause when consumed frequently.
- When consumed regularly, soya can reduce the risk of several cancers, including breast cancer.
- Soya can help protect against heart disease and osteoporosis and help with weight loss.
- Starting soya in childhood or as a young adult has even more benefits.
- There is no need to avoid soya if you are on thyroid medications but be aware of meal timing.
- Soya is best eaten in the minimally processed form, such as edamame beans, tofu, tempeh, and soya milk.
- Two–four portions of soya are recommended daily (80 g is one portion).

15

Stronger with age: Ensuring adequate protein by Rohini Bajekal, Nutritionist

Rohini Bajekal, nutritionist

Protein has an essential role to play in human health. There are several times in a woman's life where a higher protein intake is important, including perimenopause and menopause. Of all the macronutrients, it is clear that protein gets the most hype. Over the years, both fat and carbohydrates have been vilified in turn, but protein has generally escaped this public reckoning. However, there are many myths surrounding protein, leading to a great deal of confusion around the optimal amount and the best sources. There are other aspects of nutrition to consider too, including the fact that energy requirements decrease as we age, as the result of a reduced basal metabolic rate. Therefore, the quality and composition of our diet become especially important during this chapter of life.

The role of protein

Protein, as a component of muscle and bone, is essential for our body's structure and movement. Protein is made up of many building blocks, known as amino acids. There are 20 different amino acids that the body needs to function properly. Some of these amino acids can be produced by the body, while nine of these amino acids must be obtained from our diet. These are known as essential amino acids. Protein is needed for the growth, maintenance and repair of body tissues, healthy muscles, and strong bones. It also plays a crucial role in healthy immune function, cell signalling, and muscle and nerve contraction.

As we get older, our body's ability to utilize protein may become less efficient, so it is sensible for older adults to aim for higher protein intakes. Observational studies suggest that higher protein intakes are associated with higher lean body mass in post-menopausal women. In the Women's Health Initiative study, a higher protein intake (1.2 g per kg body weight) was associated with a 32 per cent lower risk of frailty and improved physical function.[1,2] Making this minor adjustment to the balance of macronutrients in our diet can also help with weight management, potentially helping to prevent excess weight gain as well as loss of lean muscle mass. These dietary changes do not need to be overwhelming and can be achievable with small tweaks.

While protein intake is undoubtedly important, it is most effective when combined with resistance training, which sends the signal for strong bones and maintenance of lean muscle. For the vast majority of us living in the Western world, it is most likely that loss of strength as we age is due to modern sedentary lifestyles rather than not getting enough protein in the diet.

The myth of incomplete protein

The idea that you *need* to eat foods in certain combinations to get adequate protein originated from a book published almost 50 years ago. While this has since been totally disproven, the myth prevails. In fact, all plant cells contain all nine essential amino acids, the building blocks of protein, in differing amounts. Our bodies cycle through amino acids on a daily basis so as long as we are eating a varied diet and meeting energy requirements, we will not run into major issues.

The belief that plant protein is inferior to animal protein is also very prevalent. While the protein in whole plant foods such as beans and lentils may be less digestible than meat, we can offset that by slightly increasing overall protein intake and choosing foods such as tempeh and tofu which contain highly digestible protein and a very good amount of all essential amino acids. It is important to recognize that different foods do have different proportions of amino acids. For example, most seeds and beans are lower in methionine but rich in lysine whereas grains are rich in methionine but low in lysine. While grains and beans do not need to be necessarily combined in a single meal, they often are prepared this way. For example, rice and dal, porridge with soya milk, a peanut butter sandwich or black bean tacos.

Table 1 Common plant sources of protein in the diet

	Food type	Protein content (g) per 100 g
Pulses	Red lentils (boiled)	7.6
	Chickpeas (canned)	7.2
Beans	Tofu (steamed)	8.1
	Kidney beans (canned)	6.9
	Baked beans	5.0
Grains	Wheat flour (brown)	12.2
	Rice (easy cook, boiled)	10.9
	Bread (brown)	7.9
	Bread (white)	7.9
	Pasta (dried cooked)	4.8
	Porridge oats	3.0
Nuts	Almonds	21.1
	Walnuts	14.7
	Hazelnuts	14.1

Source: Mc Cance and Widdowson's The Composition of Foods, 2015[3,4]

When we consider a food, we need to evaluate its *entire* package rather than reducing its benefit or harm to a single nutrient. Animal protein comes packaged with several undesirable characteristics such as haem iron, dietary cholesterol, and saturated fat whereas plant protein is loaded with beneficial fibre and other protective nutrients. Reflecting this, dietary guidelines around the world, including the UK, USA and Canada, promote a shift towards getting more protein from plant-based sources such as beans, peas, lentils and less from meat and meat products, particularly red and processed meats. Plant proteins also have a significant environmental advantage.

Protein needs as we get older

While most countries' guidelines differ, the European clinical guidelines for older adults recommend a protein intake of at least 1 g of protein per kg per day and around 1–1.2 g is thought to be the amount that older adults should aim for. For a 60 kg woman, this would work out to 60–72 g of protein.

It is interesting to examine what current intakes are among older adults. A study looking at protein intake in over 8000 older adults found that 22 per cent of adults aged 55 or older did not achieve the RDA of 0.8 g per kg of body weight, and 70 per cent failed to reach 1.2 g per kg, the latter of which is generally considered a more optimal protein intake for maintaining muscle and strength as we age.[5,6] This suggests that protein intakes may not be as high as we assume in older adults, despite the fact that the average intake for an American adult is 1.3 g per kg. The situation is similar in the United Kingdom. While average protein intakes in the UK are above the Reference Nutrient Intake (RNI), this may not be the case for older adults. Fewer than 50 per cent of participants in a UK study met current UK recommendations (0.75 g per kg) and fewer than 15 per cent met the 1.2 g per kg age-specific recommendation.[7] The good news is that with some dietary adjustments, it is possible to obtain these protein intakes on a plant-predominant diet without the need for any additional supplements.

The source of the protein matters

Many people equate protein only with meat, fish, dairy and eggs and automatically assume that plant-based diets must lack protein. While it is true that all plant foods contain some protein, foods such as fruit contain very little. There are however many nutritious plant-based sources of protein including tofu, tempeh, mycoprotein (fungi-based protein such as Quorn™), seitan, beans, lentils, chickpeas, peanuts, soya milk and legume pasta. These foods are far lower in saturated fat than meat as well as generally higher in fibre, vitamins and minerals and phytonutrients. Soya foods such as tofu and tempeh are particularly rich sources of protein.

Swapping calories from animal protein with calories from plant protein is also associated with a lower risk of premature death. Replacing just 3 per cent of total energy in the diet from animal protein with plant-derived protein can significantly reduce mortality from a number of causes with a risk reduction in the order of 20–40 per cent. An additional 3 per cent energy from plant proteins a day was associated with a 5 per cent lower risk of death from all causes.[8] This suggests that even smaller shifts in the direction of plant protein can have massive benefits. Choosing plant protein sources may also be associated with overall longevity. We know that plant foods reduce oxidative stress and inflammation, both of which contribute to the ageing process.

The role of protein as a bone-protective nutrient must also not be underestimated as we have seen in Chapter 5 by Dr Rajiv Bajekal. Sources of plant protein such as tofu and beans also contain other nutrients that benefit bone health such as calcium, potassium, and manganese. Higher protein intakes play a key role in healthy ageing to reduce the risk of osteoporosis and sarcopenia, as well as promoting optimal physical function.

Protein for active and busy lifestyles

While it's true that anyone who is strength training needs extra protein, appetites tend to naturally increase with activity so increasing servings of protein-rich foods at meals is a way of accounting for this. It can also be helpful to include some processed foods such as plant-based meat alternatives, textured vegetable protein (TVP), bean-based pastas, or a plant-based protein powder blend to make the diet less bulky and fibrous. It also makes it easier to hit protein targets with a weight loss or maintenance goal or for those who simply struggle to eat enough. These processed foods are by no means necessary, but they are safe providing that the foundation of the diet consists of whole grains, legumes, fruit, vegetables, nuts, and seeds. You may wish to avoid protein powders with added sweeteners, bulking agents, and fillers, which can sometimes contribute to digestive issues for those prone to this.

There has been a huge backlash around processed foods in recent years and it's clear that high consumption of ultra-processed foods has a detrimental impact on our health. However, some processed foods help us meet nutritional needs, whether it's canned beans, pre-cooked grains, or fortified soya milk. When soya beans are soaked and cooked to be turned into soya milk or tofu, they are easier to digest, and mineral availability also increases. We should not discount the importance of convenience and taste in modern day life where few of us have the time or desire to spend hours preparing meals from scratch.

Insulin resistance and protein intake

As we enter the perimenopause and menopause, many women gradually put on weight and become more insulin resistant. Insulin is the vital hormone that regulates blood sugar (glucose) in the body. Insulin resistance means that the cells of the body cannot use blood glucose as effectively, meaning that blood sugar levels can stay elevated for longer. However, even modest weight loss of between 3 and 5 per cent can lower glucose and halt the development of type 2 diabetes. Dietary and lifestyle changes can help most people to become more insulin sensitive, for example, eating more high-fibre foods, getting more sleep, reducing stress levels and so on. You can also improve insulin sensitivity by exercising, even without weight loss.

Low-carb diets are not necessarily the answer to insulin resistance. A low-carb diet claims to be high protein but is often high in meat, dairy and eggs and therefore is a high saturated fat diet, with intakes often exceeding the recommendation of staying below 10 per cent of total energy intake. Saturated fat increases insulin resistance. If you prefer a low-carb diet, the safest way of doing this is likely the Eco-Atkins diet or lower carb plant-predominant diet but do consider that these can feel restrictive for some people and health-promoting foods such as whole grains are eliminated.

Learning to make plant protein a priority

As we get older, many people, especially women, start favouring quick snacks or lighter meals rather than protein-rich options. An extreme version of this is seen in tea and toast syndrome, a form of malnutrition commonly experienced by elderly people who are unable to prepare meals and tend to themselves. Increasing access to education around nutrition and identifying healthful sources of protein can help people to make gradual changes. For example, choosing a protein-rich source at every meal or snack can be a good rule of thumb as well as learning how to cook high-protein meals.

There is no evidence-based reason to be wary of limiting protein when it is sourced from plant foods, which offer a great deal of nutritional value beyond protein content. While you do not need to obsess over your protein intake, being aware that choosing protein-rich foods at mealtimes may make your perimenopause and menopause transition easier. When possible, opt for plant-based sources of protein as these promote health and longevity, as well as delivering fibre, vitamins, minerals, and other beneficial phytonutrients. Remember to incorporate strength training and other healthy lifestyle habits so you can reap the benefits of this minor dietary adjustment.

Menopause mantra: *I will use plant-based sources to increase my protein intake*

- Enjoy at least three servings of legumes a day: soya milk/ yoghurt, beans, lentils, tofu, tempeh.
- Swap other plant milks for soya milk or pea milk.
- Consider a plant-based protein powder with blends of soya, pea, rice, and hemp protein especially if you have a weight loss goal, are strength training or find it hard to meet protein needs through your diet.
- Swap crisps or popcorn for higher-protein snacks such as roasted chickpeas, edamame or a handful of nuts.
- Switch starch-based pasta (e.g. wheat pasta or brown rice pasta) to a legume-based pasta such as edamame bean or lentil or chickpea pasta.
- Choose the most protein-rich grains and starchy foods such as potatoes, oats, amaranth and quinoa.
- Find ways to add protein into meals such as blending red lentils into a curry or silken tofu into a creamy pasta sauce.
- Include vegetables that are naturally higher in protein such as sweetcorn, broccoli, and spinach for a protein boost.
- Try toppings and dressings that are rich in some protein such as nutritional yeast, peanut butter, and hummus.

16

Eat the rainbow: Transitioning to a plant-based diet

'I've tried eating this way before and I found it too hard.'

I hear this time and time again from my patients and the women I speak to. In this chapter, I explain how to transition successfully to this way of eating. There is no one right way to make the transition but it should always be joyful and interesting.

Some people feel ready to make the shift overnight, whereas others prefer to gradually include more plant-based foods in their diet over time. The latter may give your body time to adjust to all the delicious foods you will consume, allowing your gut microbiome to adapt to the increase in fibre, and lessen side effects such as bloating and gas. This will also give you the time to educate yourself on the science backing this way of eating. I have enlisted expert nutritionist Rohini for her input into this chapter.

Making the switch

It is worth the time and effort to learn practical ways to introduce more plant-based foods into your diet when it comes to making the switch. Learning nutrition basics and the common challenges you may face can make this way of eating sustainable both in the short term but also in the long term. Once you see the many benefits to your energy levels, bloating and other aspects of your health, you will not look back.

Crowd out certain foods to let others in

As many of you may not have grown up eating a lot of plant-based foods, it takes time and education to reimagine your plate in a new way, especially coming up with meals without animal products. All healthy dietary patterns require consideration, so don't let the idea that you need to 'plan' a healthy plant-based diet overwhelm you. Crowding out animal foods and ultra-processed foods by adding in plant-based ingredients which are nutrient-dense and tasty is a good way to ensure nutrient density and satiety. This means swapping meat, dairy, fish and eggs for protein-, iron- and zinc-rich foods such as beans, lentils, tofu, tempeh and textured vegetable protein (TVP). Soya is versatile and has many health benefits for all women, including those in perimenopause and menopause.

Fill your plate with colour

Every large study confirms that a dietary pattern that is centred around whole plant foods, rich in colourful fruits and vegetables, whole grains, legumes, nuts and seeds, herbs and spices, is one of the healthiest choices you can make. Leading dietetic organizations around the world have confirmed that eating this way can meet nutritional requirements at all stages of life, from birth to old age.

Change it up

Join a cooking class or visit a restaurant that serves mouth-watering foods from the many cultures and cuisines that have been prioritizing plants for hundreds of years, such as Ethiopian, Indian, Chinese and Mexican. Most importantly, make it fun. If you don't enjoy cooking very much or don't have the time during the week, consider batch cooking on the weekend. You can then assemble colourful bowls with some key ingredients, warm and cold, to keep you feeling full and happy.

Experiment

When starting out, try not to be restrictive with your food choices. Experiment with new recipes to expand your plant-based meal repertoire and try one-pot stews, curries and colourful stir-fries. Experiment with new flavours and textures, and discover the incredible diversity that exists within plant-based eating.

It is also a good idea to try some of the newer alternatives on offer if you'd like, such as plant-based meat alternatives. These can be especially helpful when making the transition as they can provide familiarity in terms of texture and flavour, are convenient to prepare and are often fortified with key nutrients. However, where possible, aim to base most of your meals around whole plant foods which tend to be more beneficial for health, the environment and your wallet.

Practise non-judgement

It is helpful to look at food without guilt. It can take time but try to nurture a positive mindset to eating. Remember no single food has the ability to make or break your health, instead look at the bigger picture.

As you bring in changes, try not to be too hard on yourself, especially if you have not been able to sustain some of your dietary changes. Life has a habit of getting in the way and no one is perfect. Remind yourself that it's okay to slip up – an all-or-nothing thinking doesn't help.

Remember your 'Why?'

Whether you have gone plant-based for improving your health in menopause or for the environment or for the animals, it's important to remember your 'Why?' to stay on track. Some people benefit from watching documentaries about the environment, making new friends who follow the same lifestyle, or writing down their health goals to strengthen their resolve.

If you are committed to a plant-based lifestyle but need individual support, reach out to a qualified nutritionist or dietitian who understands plant-based nutrition and can guide you.

Nutrition guidance

Everyone can benefit from medical nutrition advice, but it can be especially helpful if you have a medical condition such as coeliac disease, a history of disordered eating, high blood pressure or type 2 diabetes or are finding perimenopause or menopause challenging.

Areas to focus on while transitioning

Enjoy complex carbohydrates

Enjoy mostly intact whole grains such as porridge oats, quinoa, millet, brown and red rice, as well as starchy vegetables cooked with the skin on such as sweet potatoes and potatoes. Try Chinese potatoes, Jerusalem artichokes, yams and tapiocas. Don't be scared of 'carbs'. We need them.

Eat protein-rich foods

Getting enough protein is generally not an issue if you are eating a variety of plant-based foods and getting enough calories. However, if you are excluding beans, lentils and soya from your diet or you are undereating, you are more likely to struggle. Add tofu or tempeh into stir-fries, base meals around lentils and beans. Include protein-rich ingredients in meals such as peanuts and hummus and replace dairy with fortified soya milk. Add a plant protein powder (soya or pea or brown rice protein) to smoothies before or after a workout.

Add omega 3-rich foods

Enjoy 2 tablespoons of ground flaxseed every day on your porridge or in your smoothie and include other omega 3-rich foods in your diet such as milled chia seeds, walnuts and hemp seeds. Consider an algae-derived omega 3 supplement daily.

Take a B12 supplement

It is especially important to ensure a reliable vitamin B12 supplement (oral or spray) on a plant-based diet or if you are over the age of 65 in the UK, or over age 50 in the USA and in certain other situations, whatever your diet. People are often not aware that B12 is made by the microbes in our soil, and typically added to products or supplemented in animals in factory farms.

Menopause mantra: *Eat the rainbow*

- Look forward to trying new foods.
- Fill your plate with colour.
- Crowd out certain foods to let others in.
- Experiment with different cuisines and new flavours.
- Practise non-judgement.
- Take your time.
- Remember your 'Why?'.
- Supplement with B12 and consider other key supplements.
- Make the change fun.

17

A diet for all: The link between human and planetary health

The world is finally waking up to the climate crisis, with floods, forest fires, melting glaciers, rising sea levels, and unseasonable weather firmly at our doorstep and in our backyard, with nowhere to run. Scientists have known about climate change and our role in this as humans for decades, but little has been done by countries and their governments to heed their advice, except for some half-hearted attempts to try to mitigate the looming disaster.

The earth's climate has seen unprecedented changes like never before, driven by human-induced global warming of 1.1 degrees C.[1]

The global south has been feeling the devastating effects of climate change since at least the last half-century, with floods in Bangladesh and droughts in Africa putting millions of people out of homes and driving millions more into starvation. The messaging by responsible authorities has been weak, leaving the public confused. Now that the climate emergency is upon us in the global north, there is no denying it.

Climate change is real

The IPCC (Intergovernmental Panel on Climate Change), the world's most authoritative scientific body, released an eight-year-long undertaking on 20 March 2023, based on the findings of over 700 scientists, on the physical science of climate change, impacts, adaptation and vulnerability to climate change and ways to mitigate this crisis. At around 8000 pages, this AR6 (sixth assessment report) is the most comprehensive scientific assessment of climate change to date.[2]

The AR6 details the devastating consequences of rising greenhouse gas emissions around the world, as well as the irreversible changes and collapse of communities should humans fail to act and change course.

Fossil fuels, such as oil, carbon and natural gas, are the number one source of greenhouse gas emissions with transport, power generation, industry etc. responsible for close to 80 per cent of global emissions and agriculture, forestry and other land uses for the remainder.

The AR6 report also gives us hope. If we bring in the recommended adaptative measures now, we can make for a more resilient future on our planet, helping save populations and ecosystems that have not already been completely destroyed.

Key solutions needed to mitigate climate change

There is universal agreement now that the climate crisis is real and we, as humans, are causing it.[1,2] The question to ask, therefore, is 'What can we do?' Should we resign ourselves to a ravaged planet with a bleak future awaiting our children and future generations, or is there something we can all do?

Limiting the use of fossil fuels and replacing them with renewable and cleaner sources of energy is without question something we all need to do. According to the Carbon Majors Report, just 100 companies have been responsible for more than 70 per cent of global greenhouse gas emissions over the last three decades.[3] As recommended by the IPCC, changes need to happen on an international policy level, but there are also changes we can make at an individual level. This means rethinking how we travel. Using public transport, walking and cycling wherever possible and accessible to us, switching to electric vehicles, as well as taking fewer flights and staying longer in a particular destination, are all ways for us to reduce our carbon footprint.

Eating more plants

Turns out there is also another way, one that will let us do our bit in helping the planet, and delay or maybe even avert the inevitable. It will also help our own individual health tremendously and the current health crisis and medical care system, drowning under the tsunami of chronic diseases, responsible for killing 11 million people, and harming millions more, every year worldwide.[4]

Of the ten key solutions proposed by the IPCC, one of them is to eat more plants and less meat. In other words, adopting a plant-based diet or a plant-predominant diet is not just best for human health but also the best diet for planetary health. Reducing food waste is imperative too and is another key solution.

Adopting a planetary diet

The 2019 Eat-Lancet study, involving 37 world renowned scientists from 16 countries, proposed scientific targets for what constitutes both a healthy diet and a sustainable food system. Their recommendation was for the human population to collectively move to eating a plant-predominant diet (flexitarian), with optional small amounts of animal products (71 g of meat and fish, 250 ml of dairy and 13 g of eggs in a day).[5,6,7]

The aims of the report and suggested diet are as follows:

- Feed the world's population of 10 billion people by 2050.
- Greatly reduce the worldwide number of deaths caused by poor diet.
- Be environmentally sustainable to avoid collapse of the natural world.

What we eat matters

Food is the strongest lever we have to optimize human health, while ensuring environmental sustainability on Earth.[8] An urgent transition to a plant-based food system is essential for the health of humans, non-human animals and the future of our planet. Government policies have to improve access to healthy plant-based foods, making them affordable to all. We have to demand governments stop subsidising meat and dairy which are hurting our health and the planet. Regardless of the distance from the farm to your plate, even the most sustainably produced animal foods generate more greenhouse gas emissions than any plant foods.

More antibiotics are used in animals and fish than in humans, contributing to the huge rise in the number of antibiotic-resistant infections. The United Nations has warned that an extra 10 million people may die by 2050 as a result of completely preventable antibiotic resistance.

We can be the change

Many of the people I meet genuinely want to change, but are confused or scared by what they have heard from friends or on social media. You may also be alarmed by healthcare professionals, unaware of the science themselves, who may not support your decision to go plant-based.

Choose plant-based options

Without doubt our diets should be centred around whole plant foods, but there is no need to miss out on treats, as innovation in food technology has led to tasty plant-based meat, dairy, egg and fish alternatives, without the immense environmental impact.

Compassion

Every year, a staggering 80 billion land animals are killed for food, and close to 3 trillion sea animals. The oceans that support vast ecosystems are emptying at an unimaginable pace. The accompanying animal suffering is untold.

The most wonderful thing about eating plants is that not only is a plant-based diet great for our health but also, as we have seen, best for planetary health. It is also the kindest diet for the fellow beings we share our beautiful home with. We should be able to look at future generations and say, 'We tried our best'.

There are many reliable resources, including my nutritious recipes, which you can access (Part 4) to help you on your plant-based adventure. *You can do it.*

Menopause mantra: *I can make a difference*

- What's on our plates matters at many levels.
- Climate change is real, with communities and ecosystems close to collapse.
- Adopt a planetary diet (plant-predominant).
- Reduce meat, dairy and other animal products significantly in your diet.
- A planetary diet is the best both for human health and planetary health.
- A planetary diet can create a sustainable food system to feed the world's population.
- Minimize food and water waste.
- Use public transport, walk and bike where possible, switch to electric vehicles.
- Take fewer flights and stay longer if you do fly to mitigate effects.
- A planetary diet is kinder to the sentient beings we share this beautiful planet with.

18

Empty promises: The truth about most supplements

The global market for dietary supplements is booming, valued at USD 167.8 billion in 2019, and is expected to hit a record value of USD 306.8 billion by 2026. It is not unusual for my patients to bring out at least ten different supplements they are taking hoping for relief with their menopausal symptoms, whether it is for their hot flushes, for weight loss, to improve skin, reduce hair loss or manage joint aches.

The overwhelming majority of expensive supplements taken by women in the hope of seeing improvement of their symptoms are in fact not going to keep the promise on the label and may in some situations cause harm. At the very least, even when effects are neutral, it is a waste of money which is better spent on high quality food, a massage or even a holiday.

I empathize with women who are often struggling with their menopausal symptoms, worried (falsely) about taking HRT, so turn to supplements for menopause and hormonal health, believing unsubstantiated claims with little evidence to back them and surrounded by marketing hype.

Food first

It is important to appreciate that supplements can never replace eating a diverse and varied plant-predominant diet. The food and drink we consume on a daily basis affect our hormonal and general health. Plant foods contain thousands of beneficial micronutrients such as carotenoids, flavonoids, and polyphenols, as well as essential vitamins, minerals, fibre and water, which are difficult to encapsulate in a single or even a few supplements.

Special situations

There are a few situations where we may not be able to obtain all our nutrients from food and different variables may be at play. These include pregnancy, certain medical conditions or medications that hinder absorption, limited access to healthy foods, allergies and intolerances, soil quality and even how much sunlight we get. Supplements do have a role to play in these situations.

A note of caution: It is important for you to mention to your doctor which supplements you take, as these may interact with the medications prescribed, altering their effects or causing harm to you. An individualized approach is advised if supplements are to be added for menopause, ideally with the help of a qualified health professional.

The role of supplements in perimenopause and menopause

There are certain supplements most women should be taking for optimal health. For the rest of the supplements that I mention, there is little robust scientific evidence to recommend routine use.

Vitamin D

Vitamin D is a fat-soluble vitamin and as its synthesis occurs in our skin on exposure to sunlight, it is technically a hormone. Sunlight is very variable depending on where you live, and cannot be relied on for vitamin D synthesis completely. Food sources such as eggs and mushrooms are also unreliable, due to insufficient and variable amounts. Vitamin D is needed for bone and neurological health, maintaining calcium balance in the blood and for the immune system. Vitamin D deficiency is common in women worldwide, and can worsen immunity and insulin resistance.

After an initial blood test to measure levels, the advisable dosage of vitamin D3 can vary between 400–2000 IU/day taken with the largest meal of the day, ideally throughout the year, but especially in the winter months. If higher doses are needed, they should be used only under medical guidance to avoid vitamin D toxicity.

In addition to supplementing, direct sunshine between the hours of 11 am to 3 pm on your arms, legs or back for 15–45 minutes, depending on the colour of your skin, can help you produce your vitamin D; 30–45 minutes are needed for darker skin. Apply an adequate amount of recommended sunscreen (SPF 50 ideally) to reduce the risk of skin cancer. Choose a mineral sunscreen over standard sunscreens, as there appears to be better protection from ultraviolet radiation, checking it is approved as UVA (EU standard).

Vitamin B12

Vitamin B12 (cobalamin) is a water-soluble vitamin and essential nutrient which helps keep the body's nerve and blood cells healthy and plays a role in forming DNA (the genetic material in all cells). Vitamin B12 deficiency may take several years to manifest as the body has stores which last a while, and symptoms can range from fatigue to permanent neurological damage. Vitamin B12 deficiency can also cause a type of anaemia known as megaloblastic anaemia. Independent of the anaemia, B12 deficiency can damage the nervous system, which is serious.

A note of caution: This supplement is essential if you are on a plant-based diet at any age. On any diet, supplementation is recommended in people above the age of 50 in the USA and above age 65 in the UK, as gastric absorption of B12 tends to reduce with age.

Vitamin B12 dosage

It is a good idea to take a Vitamin B12 supplement of at least 50 mcg–100 mcg daily, and 1000 mcg daily if you are over the age of 65. Choose cyanocobalmin where possible, as it is more shelf-stable and cheaper than methylcobalamin.

The recommended daily intake (RDI) of vitamin B12 is 2.4 mcg for both men and women. As only 10 mcg of a 500 mcg B12 supplement is absorbed in people without a deficiency, there is a need for higher supplement doses than the body's daily needs of the vitamin.

Vitamin B12 is better absorbed in smaller, frequent doses. This is because B12 binds to a substance called intrinsic factor released in the stomach. This process is easily overwhelmed if there is one big dose, rather than divided over two separate meals. Only enough intrinsic factor is excreted per meal to absorb 2–4 mcg of B12.

If you choose to obtain B12 from enriched foods, like yeast extract, fortified meat alternatives or nutritional yeast, then a serving will need to be eaten at least twice a day for the same reason. I would still recommend a supplement of B12, as the neurological side effects of vitamin B12 deficiency can be dangerous and sometimes irreversible.

Vitamin B12 injections raise levels quicker and may be needed if a deficiency is diagnosed. Some people cannot absorb Vitamin B12 due to certain digestive conditions and therefore need injections under the guidance of a health professional.

Vitamin B12 supplements are generally safe but too high a dose may cause side effects such as dizziness, headaches, nausea, and vomiting. Vitamin B12 supplements can also interact with other drugs such as metformin for diabetes and vitamin C among others, so it is wise to check with your doctor if in any doubt.

It is a good idea to get your vitamin B12 and vitamin D levels checked at least once a year.

Iodine

Iodine is a trace element and an essential component of our thyroid hormones. The daily requirement of iodine is about 140 mcg and if you are concerned you are not getting the required amount in your diet, you may wish to take a supplement. Too much iodine can be a problem just as too little can.

Salt in the UK is not iodized, and neither are rock salts. Seaweed and sea vegetables such as nori and dulse are good iodine sources, but they contain varying amounts and can be unreliable. Iodized salt is also a good source, but we have already discussed how one should try to minimize salt in general. In some people, overconsumption of raw cruciferous vegetables may block the thyroid gland's ability to absorb iodine.

Iron

If you are having heavy or frequent periods in perimenopause, seek medical advice soon. A blood test will guide your doctor to advise you if you need iron supplements. One in five women who suffer from iron deficiency anaemia do so because of heavy periods. Treating the underlying cause along with an iron-rich diet (legumes, tofu, green leafy vegetables, apricots, cashew nuts for example) and iron supplements will treat your iron deficiency. If you are not having periods or bleeding from any other site and blood tests show you are not low in iron, you do not need to take routine iron supplements.

Omega 3 fatty acids

These are a type of polyunsaturated fat. They are essential fats, which means our body cannot make them on its own and we need them to survive as they are involved throughout the body at a cellular level and are important for brain health. We get the omega 3 fatty acids we need from the foods we eat.

The form of omega 3 in plants is called alpha-linolenic acid (ALA) and is needed to make other two omega 3 fats. These other two important long chain fatty acids that have the most direct health benefits are eicosapentaenoic acid (EPA) and docosahexaenoic acid (DHA). They are found in algae and plankton which are eaten by fish; hence fish is a rich source of EPA and DHA. Fish per se does not make omega 3 as is commonly believed. Avoid fish liver oil supplements because of the higher content of heavy metals such as mercury.

Omega 3-rich foods

As some people don't convert ALA from food substances very efficiently, it may be worth considering an algae-derived omega 3 supplement (EPA and DHA) of 1000 mg daily, especially as one gets older. In addition, consider including 1–2 tablespoons of milled flaxseed powder daily and/or 1 teaspoon chia seeds (soaked) daily and/or 6 walnut halves daily and/or ¼ cup hemp seeds, all good sources of ALA.

Supplements in perimenopause and menopause in general are not needed other than the ones discussed above.

Isoflavone supplements

While some trials have shown a reduction in hot flushes using isoflavone supplements (soya, red clover or lignans such as flaxseed), a review of all literature suggests these isoflavone supplements are no better than a placebo or have a weak and variable action.[1,2,3]

Isoflavones are a type of phytoestrogens or plant oestrogens. Of the isoflavones that seem to have the most benefit in the reduction of hot flushes is daidzein, found in soya. Unlike dietary consumption of soya which is safe and beneficial in those with breast cancer (see Chapter 14), experts suggest caution in taking these supplements until more evidence is available regarding their safety. My advice is to try to stay away from isoflavone supplements found in many expensive supplements marketed as the 'magic bullet' for menopausal symptoms.

I always recommend eating soya in the form of tofu, tempeh, edamame beans and soya milk. It is more affordable, safer, and better for you as it comes with the added protein, fibre, and micronutrients. Try drinking sage leaf or raspberry leaf tea, which contain flavonoids and may help menopausal symptoms as part of your diet, and 2 tbsp daily of milled flaxseed on your porridge or in your smoothie, rich in omega 3 fatty acids and lignans that may regulate oestrogen levels and hot flushes.

Botanical or herbal supplements

Look for the THR logo standing for traditional herbal medicines that have been approved for their dosage, quality and product information, as most herbal medications are unregulated with unpredictable doses and purity. Black cohosh is probably one of the most popular (second to isoflavone supplements) for managing hot flushes. A review of all available literature suggests that black cohosh is no more effective than a placebo for hot flushes. In general, black cohosh is safe, although some caution is advised in breast cancer. Black cohosh may cause mild drug interactions with certain medications such as tamoxifen, a drug used in breast cancer, and was previously thought to affect liver function, but this does not appear to be the case on review of studies.[1]

Chinese herbs such as wild yam and dong quai for treatment of hot flushes have not been shown to be effective from available studies.[1,4]

Maca, a member of the brassica family, native to South America, pollen extract, and evening primrose oil also cannot be recommended routinely due to lack of evidence for managing menopausal symptoms. Similarly, lemon balm, vitex agnus castus, gingko biloba, liquorice, fennel, valerian and other medicinal plants have been studied and may be effective in managing vasomotor symptoms of menopause through different mechanisms, but the scientific evidence is weak for any to be recommended routinely.[4]

St John's wort has been shown to improve mild to moderate depression in the general population and may help with mood changes seen in women approaching menopause.[5,6]

Collagen supplements for skin and joints

Collagen makes up about one-third of the body's protein and provides support for our skin, muscles, bones and joints. You may have heard a lot of hype around collagen supplements, much more than what the scientific evidence suggests. Taking a supplement of collagen needs it to be broken down and reassembled, hence it does not translate into a direct increase in your collagen levels. Collagen supplements contain amino acids, the building blocks of protein, and may have added zinc, biotin, vitamin C etc., and are usually derived from bovine or marine sources. Larger trials are needed before experts will advise taking these expensive supplements. In the meantime, having a diet rich in legumes, tofu, green leafy vegetables, citrus fruits, using sunscreen, avoiding smoking and regular exercise can all help your body make collagen naturally and improve skin.

Probiotics for gut and vaginal health

Taking oral probiotics, which are in effect a few colonies of healthy bacteria instead of the trillions of organisms that make up the gut microbiome, is found to be of limited benefit in general. Probiotics should only be prescribed, ideally for a short period, under the guidance of a qualified health professional, as they may over time displace the other healthy bacteria. There may be a case for a course of medically approved probiotics, if you have certain medical conditions or are on a prolonged course of antibiotics, otherwise the case is currently weak for probiotics.

The best prebiotics and probiotics come from whole plant foods. Eating a diverse and varied plant-predominant diet can help the healthy gut and vaginal microbiome to flourish, without resorting to expensive shop-bought probiotics. Focus on adding more fruit, vegetables, beans, soya, herbs and spices, garlic, nuts and seeds, fermented foods such as sauerkraut, pickled vegetables, kimchi into your daily diet, as these provide the food or the prebiotics for the healthy bacteria (probiotics) to feast on and multiply.

Tell your doctor

Despite the fact that there is limited scientific evidence confirming that they work and that they are safe, many women find these 'natural treatments' appealing, often preferring them to regulated menopausal hormone therapy (HRT). Three-quarters of women do not tell their doctor about the supplements they take, partly because they are not asked, and also because medical doctors are unfamiliar with the alternative options that their patients may be choosing without their knowledge.

Menopause mantra: *I will choose supplements carefully alongside a food-first approach*

- There is a lack of robust evidence to support most herbal and botanical supplements in reducing hot flushes in menopause. Look for the THR logo if choosing these.
- A food-first approach is advised for most women before expensive menopause supplements.
- Vitamin D and vitamin B12 supplements are recommended.
- Iron supplements may be needed for women in perimenopause with heavy periods.
- Probiotics are not helpful except in select situations.
- Collagen supplements are not recommended.
- Inform your doctor if you are on supplements as they may interact with your medications.

19

Menopause movement: Physical activity and exercise

Growing up in Kolkata at a time when girls were meant to be seen and not heard, let alone wear shorts and run around with boys, I was fortunate that my parents encouraged me to be active. I competed in track and field events, and played basketball right through school and college, enjoying almost any form of exercise. I also walked everywhere, as we didn't have a car until we came to the UK, aged 30.

However, the long hours as a junior doctor in India, and subsequently in the UK, soon put paid to any structured exercise, as time off was used to catch up on sleep or do research. Getting 10,000 steps daily, however, was easy for me. Ask any hospital doctor in an acute specialty like Obstetrics and Gynaecology. Those steps add up in no time, as we have to be on our feet often more than 12 hours a day, running all over the hospital attending to patients.

Except for the occasional dog walk, household chores, a young family and a full-time career meant it was almost two decades after medical school before I took up running again and going to the gym. Despite the long gap, I was able to get fit again relatively quickly, possibly because of my earlier fitness levels, and the fact that I did not have a desk job.

Numerous studies have shown that being physically active can boost both physical and mental health. Sedentary behaviours (defined as activities during waking hours in a seated or reclined position, with energy expenditure less than 1.5 times resting metabolic rate) have been shown to have adverse health impacts. We have become progressively more sedentary in the UK and US over the last 100 years, similar to many other high- and mid-income countries.

The way we work and relax, and the advent of modern technologies mean that many of us spend significant parts of our waking hours sitting in front of a screen. We do need to find a way to become more active as a population, as lack of exercise puts one in four people at risk of heart disease, type 2 diabetes, and some cancers.[1] Close to 40 per cent of women are not meeting the WHO physical activity guidelines and of all groups and genders, British women of South Asian heritage are the least likely to exercise.[2,3]

Even moving for 15 minutes a day can lower death rates. A large study of over 400,000 women and men found those who exercised at least 15 minutes a day had a 14 per cent reduced risk of all-cause mortality, and a three-year longer life expectancy compared to those who were inactive.[4]

The difference between physical activity and exercise

Physical activity is any bodily movement, however simple, that involves your muscles and helps you expend energy. Examples include climbing stairs, walking the dog leisurely or household chores. Exercise, on the other hand, is physical activity that is planned, structured and repetitive. Examples include brisk walking, swimming, jogging, Pilates and strength training. The intention with structured exercise is to improve or maintain physical fitness, strengthen the muscles and bones of your body, stabilise your joints and improve endurance through better functional health (heart and lung).

Benefits of exercise in menopause

Many of the symptoms of the perimenopause and menopause may be navigated more easily when one adds in regular exercise. It does not have to be a tough workout in the gym – you could go for a brisk walk, swim, dance, skip, do yoga, resistance training or a home workout. It doesn't matter what you do as long as you move. The best exercise is the one you enjoy. If you enjoy a particular physical activity, you are more likely to stick with it.

It should come as no surprise, however, that there is a paucity of high-quality research or large studies into the effects of exercise on hormonal health, and on women in perimenopause and menopause. Regardless of this, there is enough robust scientific evidence to suggest exercise is beneficial for all ages, and for women at all stages of their lives.

Anti-ageing

Exercise works at the cellular level, increasing the activity and number of mitochondria or 'batteries' in our cells, staving off the natural ageing process that we think is inevitable. Both external (environmental and social) and internal (genetic and biological) factors contribute to inflammation, the foundation for the development of chronic diseases, and ultimately responsible for the functional decline in our body cells and tissues.

Any intervention that can reduce chronic inflammation may help slow cellular ageing. These include changes in diet and lifestyle. Many of the anti-ageing effects of exercise may be by modulating intracellular signalling, and through activating certain enzymes such as AMPK (5' adenosine monophosphate-activated protein kinase), known as the body's master regulator of energy metabolism. Drugs using these mechanisms amongst others are being developed in the hope of extending lifespan and reducing ageing.[5]

The earlier one incorporates physical movement and exercise into one's regular routine, the bigger seem to be the longer-term benefits. Even if you are a newcomer to exercise you will still reap the rewards whatever age you start. In fact, a study looking at high-intensity interval training (HIIT) was associated with an impressive 69 per cent increase in mitochondrial function in the older group, compared to 49 per cent increase in a younger group. High-intensity biking in this study effectively seemed to reverse age-related decline in mitochondrial function.[6]

Body composition

Women tend to lose muscle mass and gain abdominal fat in the years around menopause, making perimenopause perhaps the most opportune window for lifestyle interventions, including exercise.[2]

Studies have shown that both diet and intensive exercise intervention can significantly reduce the incidence of metabolic syndrome. A health impact study on perimenopausal women published in 2022 found adding intensive resistance exercise to health education and dietary guidance improved the body composition of these women, when compared to those groups receiving just health education and/or dietary guidance. The body fat and waist circumference were significantly reduced, and skeletal muscle weight significantly increased in this group.[7,8] This is encouraging news to help motivate us to add resistance training to our exercise regime.

Blood sugar regulation

This can become an issue as women tend to carry more weight in the midsection as they approach menopause. A family history of type 2 diabetes can increase one's risk of **prediabetes** and diabetes, while regular exercise can reduce the risk. Exercise can help regulate your insulin and glucose levels. Strength training is particularly helpful in making our tissues more sensitive to the action of insulin, and improve insulin resistance. It's beneficial to go for a 10–15-minute walk or do some moderate exercises after a meal for blood sugar regulation and to improve insulin resistance.

Heart disease

Exercise has been shown in several studies to improve heart health, reduce the risk of coronary artery disease, stroke, improving blood flow, making blood vessels less stiff and lowering blood pressure. This is important, as more women die of heart disease than men, and it is in fact ten times more common than breast cancer, yet most women are not aware of these facts.

Mood changes

Mood changes are common in the perimenopause and early menopause as hormones may fluctuate for years. A shift towards increased sedentary behaviour, and decreased physical activity, commonly seen in women during this phase in life, may be partly responsible for the negative impact of menopause on mental wellbeing.

Any form of exercise will help to increase the happy hormones known as endorphins (neurotransmitters), making you feel better about yourself, which in turn makes it easier for you to meet other health goals. Exercising in natural light, particularly in winter, can help banish the blues and reduce seasonal affective disorder (SAD) or winter depression. Both medium and high levels of physical activity at any stage of menopause have been found to be related to better mental well being, particularly to fewer depressive symptoms, higher levels of satisfaction with life, and a more positive attitude.[9]

Brain health

Brain health also improves with exercise, which may be attributed to the increased levels of BDNF (brain-derived neurotrophic factor). Walking has been found to increase blood flow to the brain, which is linked to better cognitive function and improved memory. Walking backwards, when done safely, has benefits of improving balance and gait, while helping challenge our brain. Physically active adults have a lower risk of cognitive decline and dementia. Managing hypertension (blood pressure) and diabetes through a combination of exercise and diet with prescribed medications as needed will further lower the risk of dementia.

Maintaining muscle and bone

This is critical to prevent falls, reduce osteoporosis and prevent muscle wasting or sarcopenia as Dr Rajiv Bajekal explains in great detail, in the chapter on bone health. Bone loss starts in our 30s with menopause further accelerating the process, so ensuring healthy muscles and bones with a healthy diet rich in whole plant foods, avoiding alcohol and smoking while building muscle and bone through resistance training will stand us in good stead as we get older.

Cancer risk

The risk of certain lifestyle-related cancers (breast, bowel, womb, ovarian and prostate for men) is lower in those who exercise regularly. Mechanisms for this reduction in cancer risk include lowering chronic inflammation, the building block of chronic illnesses, keeping body weight under control, improving immunity and reducing excess levels of oestrogen and insulin. Exercise speeds digestion, which may reduce the time that potentially harmful substances are in the colon, reducing bowel cancer risk. Exercise also lowers the risk of many of these cancers recurring.

Skin changes

Skin changes associated with menopause may be slowed with regular exercise by improving collagen levels. A 2023 study showed resistance training can counteract skin ageing such as deteriorations in skin elasticity, upper dermal structure and dermal thickness.[10] Aerobic exercise has a similar anti-ageing effect.[11,12]

Exercising to lose weight

This usually leads to frustration. We will have to exercise for several hours a day to achieve weight loss from exercise and this can be counterproductive to your health. Exercise is great for a number of things, including preventing weight gain, weight maintenance, toning and muscle building, but not specifically for weight loss.

Avoid exercising to 'cancel out calories' as this can lead to an unhealthy relationship both with food and exercise. Realizing that exercise can help improve mood, build muscle and bone, reduce cancer risk, improve hormonal, heart and brain health in menopause is much more empowering.

Period pain

Pain during periods tends to be less intense when a woman exercises regularly. Pain-inducing chemicals released from the lining of the womb, such as prostaglandins, are washed away quicker by improving blood flow through exercise, lowering the intensity of period pains. Studies have shown exercising three times a week in the run up to a period for about 45 minutes can be particularly beneficial for period pain.[13] Women in perimenopause may notice worsening period pains due to conditions such as adenomyosis (deep internal endometriosis), endometriosis, fibroids or pelvic inflammatory disease. Although exercise may help, period pain is not normal, and neither are heavy periods. My advice is not to simply accept this as a normal part of perimenopause, and to seek medical advice. Simple tests such as a pelvic ultrasound scan and blood tests can often shed a lot of light on the underlying cause, so you can have the right medical treatment.

Menopausal symptoms and the effect of exercise

The North American Menopause Society (NAMS) published a detailed systematic review in 2023 which found resistance muscle training to improve post-menopausal symptoms, including hot flush frequency, bone mineral density, fat mass and functional capacity, when compared with no exercise. When compared with aerobic exercises, resistance training may result in a reduction of hot flush frequency.[14,15,16]

There is some good research available to confirm the positive effects of exercise on the physical and psychological quality of life (QoL) scores in women with menopausal symptoms. Yoga seems to significantly improve physical QoL scores but no other menopause specific scores. Moderate-intensity aerobic exercise may result in small improvements in sleep quality and insomnia in midlife sedentary women.[14,15]

My advice is for you to work out for yourself whether your perimenopausal and menopausal symptoms are helped or made worse by a particular type of exercise and do more or less of that, remembering the other wonderful benefits of all forms of exercise and trying to do a range of different physical activities.

Exercise recommendations in perimenopause and menopause

Aim to exercise for 30–60 minutes a day, that is at least half an hour every day and ideally one hour a day. Adults need 150 to 300 minutes of moderate-intensity aerobic activity each week plus 30 minutes of muscle-strengthening activities on two days each week to get maximum health benefits from physical activity as per the NHS, WHO, CDC and USA Health and Human Services guidelines.

Types of exercise in the perimenopause and menopause should ideally include aerobic (cardiovascular exercise), strength training and flexibility as each have their own benefits.

- Swimming is an aerobic exercise and may be particularly helpful around menopause when hormones fluctuate, helping ease menopausal symptoms such as hot flushes. Cold water swimming is becoming more popular in women going through menopause. It is not just for the camaraderie, but many of the women I have spoken to say they are finding relief in some of their menopausal symptoms, as well as noticing reduced stress and better immunity. There are no robust studies yet, but there may be possible protection against dementia, protecting against brain cell death. I am not a very confident swimmer, but loved the early morning swim in the cold sea in Greystones, Ireland, with my wonderful friends, Dave and

Steve Flynn (better known as The Happy Pear; be sure to check out their recipes in this book and the Happy Menopause online course I did with them).

- Aerobic exercises such as dancing, cycling, skipping and walking briskly improve heart and lung health, build stamina and promote blood flow to your muscles. Exercising in nature can also improve our gut health and the gut microbiome. Breathe in the fresh air to improve your respiratory microbiome.

- Resistance or strength exercises such as weight training or using elastic resistance bands will help you build muscle mass, promote bone growth and provide stability to your joints. There is good evidence to show that resistance training is associated with a reduced risk of all-cause mortality, death from cardiovascular disease, and cancer-specific mortality, with a risk reduction by as much as 27 per cent when 60 minutes per week of resistance training was undertaken.[17] The recommendation of two 30-minute sessions of resistance training per week is for you to avail yourself of this extraordinary benefit.[18]

- Flexibility exercises are often underrated but stretching, Pilates, yoga and tai chi will all improve flexibility and reduce your risk of injury and falls, while enhancing balance and improving posture. Add these into your exercise routine at any age but especially as you grow older.

'Fasting or fed?'

Whether you should eat before you undertake exercise is a question that is often debated. Most studies have been not done specifically looking at women considering the varying hormonal stages, even within a single menstrual cycle, let alone in perimenopause and menopause.[19]

When it comes to women, while there are no large-scale studies, there is growing evidence to suggest exercising in a fasted state may not be advisable with regards to hormonal health.[20]

Kisspeptin, a neuropeptide or chemical messenger, plays an important role in puberty and reproduction by initiating the release of gonadotropin-releasing hormones (GnRH) from the hypothalamus, the main link between our endocrine system and the nervous system. Kisspeptin production by the hypothalamus appears to be decreased in the presence of fasting, which in turn can disrupt the release of reproductive hormones, oestrogen and progesterone. For women, exercising in the fasted state can further reduce kisspeptin, worsening hormone regulation and glucose metabolism while raising cortisol levels, causing anxiety and sleep disturbances and suppressing the thyroid.[20] Both intermittent fasting and ketogenic diets also seem to disrupt kisspeptin production.

While it does come down to personal opinion, I would much rather you had something to eat, even if it is just a banana and some peanut butter or a small smoothie, before undertaking exercise.

Helping yourself

From all the information shared above, you can see the scientific benefits of exercising and physical activity in improving hormonal health for women approaching menopause and later on in life. Regular exercise is especially important if you have a history of cancer or chronic lifestyle diseases such as type 2 diabetes or hypertension.

Once you find an exercise that you enjoy, move your body for at least half an hour a day. Aerobic exercises like dancing, brisk walking, running, elliptical training increase your heart rate and help improve your cardiovascular health, lowering your blood pressure, lipid levels and the risk of heart attack and stroke. Morning exercise routines can be good for your circadian rhythm and may help you sleep better, although any time of day is fine if mornings are inconvenient. Strength or resistance training at least twice a week has several benefits for bone, brain and metabolic health.

The North American Menopause Society (NAMS) recommends interval training for women around menopause, which incorporates exercise at a healthy rate, then increasing intensity for a short sprint, then repeating.[21] An example would be walking for five minutes, then jogging for one minute, then walking again, repeating the minute of jogging for several intervals, raising your heart rate and improving your functional capacity. If you find your vasomotor symptoms, particularly hot flushes, are worse with any kind of high-intensity interval training then I suggest you do other forms of exercise, such as swimming or maybe brisk walking (meaning you can talk, but cannot sing), which is one of the simplest aerobic exercises for menopause that you can do, and it is free.

Mix up your exercise regime for maximum health benefits and to avoid boredom. Do a variety of cardio, strength and flexibility exercises to keep healthy and consciously incorporate balance and posture exercises.

Weekend warrior

You can do all your exercise on the weekend if you do not have time but remember even 1–2 minutes of high-intensity bursts are very useful for heart health. Exercising in 10–15-minute spurts on a daily basis if you are travelling or are pressed for time is perfectly acceptable.

In your daily routine, think what you can do to move more and sit less, perhaps a standing desk for work or stretching and walking around every hour or a few squats.

Start slow and build up over time if you are not used to exercising. I always recommend getting medical advice if you are in any doubt about your medical fitness, or have an underlying medical condition, before undertaking any exercise that you are not used to.

If you can afford it, join a group exercise class where you can meet friends or likeminded people or have one-to-one sessions with a qualified personal trainer to reach your fitness potential. I suggest building up over time to an hour of moderate-intensity exercise per day five days of the week, along with a couple of sessions of muscle-strengthening exercises per week.

It is important to set realistic, achievable, and specific goals, for example, commit to a daily 20–30-minute walk with a local friend or a yoga class after work, rather than just having vague goals of 'I will exercise more' or 'I will eat better'. Build on your goals as you achieve greater levels of fitness. Finding an exercise buddy can make a real difference and helps keep you committed.

Of all the lifestyle pillars, experts agree on the benefits of exercise for all ages, with no real controversy, unlike the nutrition pillar. There are so many exercises that are free or low cost for you to choose from that you may enjoy, helping to maximize your health in menopause. Over a period of time, you will build exercise into a habit and get stronger. You will hopefully find you miss your exercise routine when you don't do it.

Physical activity and exercise

- Being physically active can boost both physical and mental health at all ages.
- Exercise has many health benefits in the menopause including reducing osteoporosis, heart disease, dementia and cancer risk.
- Exercise, both aerobic and strength training, can help with many menopausal symptoms.
- Even moving for 15 minutes a day can lower death rates.
- Exercise is anti-ageing.
- Exercise along with diet can help with improving body composition in menopause.
- Exercising after eating is better than exercising in the fasted state for hormonal health.
- 150 to 300 minutes of moderate-intensity aerobic activity each week is recommended.
- You should include 30 minutes of muscle strengthening activities on 2 days each week in addition.

Menopause mantra: *I will move my body for 30 minutes every day*

- Find an exercise you enjoy.
- Start slowly and build up over time if not used to exercise.
- Try to find an exercise buddy.
- Mix it up by doing a mixture of cardio, strength and flexibility exercises.
- Balance and posture exercises are important as one grows older.
- Seek medical advice before exercising if unsure about fitness level.
- 10–15-minute spurts and even 1–2-minute bursts also count ('exercise snacking').

20

Rested: The importance of sleep

I'll sleep when I'm dead. This was what I truly believed for a long time. How wrong I was to think I was smarter than nature. I should have known better than to question her carefully thought out and deliberate evolution design for us as humans to need sleep if we are to function at all.

My attitude to sleep was mostly due to the long hours my specialty demands, and partly because I was young and busy. A 24-hour day was often not enough, so I did what a lot of women do, I cut back on sleep. I am sure many of you can identify with this.

Like many working in the health sector or other industries such as security, hospitality, retail, or transport, I had to cope with years of disturbed sleep because of frequent night shifts. I had perfectly honed the art of sleeping through any amount of noise, waking up in a matter of seconds when the emergency bleep went off to rush to deliver a baby in difficulty or help stop pregnancy-related bleeding.

Missing even a single night's sleep can be similar to being drunk on alcohol, increasing the risk of medical errors and road traffic accidents, with studies showing being awake for 24 hours has similar effects to having a blood alcohol level higher than the UK legal limit for drivers.

I remember on one occasion desperately wanting to catch up on sleep after a 72-hour weekend from hell. Rajiv was at work and childcare was expensive. In the early 1990s, doctors didn't get the day off after a weekend of work in the UK. I had picked up our two daughters from nursery, but was desperate to have a nap before fixing their dinner. I locked the bedroom and gathered some colouring books, knowing they could not run away or harm themselves. I woke up an hour later with a start, feeling refreshed but sticky. The girls had emptied the entire contents of a large tub of thick white body cream on to the exposed parts of my face, arms and legs as they had got bored of colouring. I couldn't stop laughing – it was the best sleep I had snatched in a long time.

The importance of sleep

The amount and quality of sleep are both critical for good health for everyone. One can go for weeks without eating food, days without drinking water but sleep – try going without any for a couple of days, and I guarantee even the calmest and most rational of humans will become a gibbering wreck. No wonder sleep deprivation is considered a form of torture.

Amount of sleep

How much sleep one needs is difficult to quantify for a particular individual as it varies in the same person at different stages of their life. The American Academy of Sleep Medicine (AASM) and the Sleep Research Society recommend that adults sleep seven or more hours per night on a regular basis to promote optimal health.

Good quality sleep

Good quality sleep is essential for cell and DNA repair, fear extinguishing, memory building and information organization. Adequate sleep is needed to keep our brains healthy, improving our attention span and concentration when awake. When we sleep, our brain clears the junk material that has collected over the day, including amyloid, a fatty deposit and one of the likely markers of Alzheimer's disease. Our blood pressure and heart rate drop when we sleep at night, helping to keep our heart healthy.

Sleep is also needed to help maintain a healthy body weight by regulating cortisol levels, appetite, blood sugar and blood pressure levels, while helping us make better choices when it comes to food, alcohol and exercise. A good night's sleep helps with reducing stress levels, lowering inflammation and improving immunity, fighting off infections better. Finally, sleep is important for maintaining our relationships, for better mood and for our mental health. *With so many benefits, prioritizing sleep is essential for every one of us.*

Sleep problems

- Melatonin, an important hormone secreted by the tiny pineal gland in our brain, needs to be suppressed in the daytime, which is why exposure to morning light helps. Melatonin starts to increase closer to bedtime, but cannot do so if we are still exposed to bright lights as we near bedtime. Hence the advice to avoid blue lights from phones, tablets and computer screens if one is to have a restful night's sleep.

- Circadian disruption occurs when sleep patterns are disturbed as a result of night shift work, being exposed to light during normal sleeping hours or travel across multiple time zones. This disruption of sleep routine can have multiple health risks if it continues over an extended period of time.
- Sleep insufficiency is when a person is not getting enough restful sleep, often because of a number of factors outside their control contributing to this. Women may be working long hours, having to care for children and other family members, have hormonal health issues or other medical problems that stop them getting a full night's sleep.
- **Insomnia** is defined as 'difficulty in falling asleep, early waking, staying asleep or non-restorative sleep despite the opportunity to sleep'. Insomnia is different from sleep insufficiency, although the effects can be similar. Insomnia is thought to affect about a third of people in Western countries at least once a week and results in impaired daytime functioning. Insomnia affects women twice as much as men. Common causes of insomnia are stress, anxiety and depression. Insomnia is also a core symptom of menopause.

Hormones and sleep

Poor sleep, either from sleep insufficiency or insomnia, is seen mostly in women of all ages and stages of life, with a detrimental effect on several aspects of physical, mental, sexual, and emotional health.

Restful sleep

Restful sleep is needed for hormonal health. Women tend to suffer from sleep disturbances more than men, which is likely to be in part due to the fluctuations in oestrogen and progesterone (as well as cortisol) that occur throughout our menstrual cycle, during menstruation, in pregnancy, postpartum and in perimenopause and menopause. The feeling of a fuzzy brain, fatigue, tiredness, instead of feeling refreshed on waking up, is real for many women at several stages in their lives, including around menopause.

Hormonal fluctuations

These can be experienced by women in perimenopause, and early years of menopause, and can lead to a disturbed sleep pattern, which in turn worsens premenstrual symptoms before a period, as well as hot flushes and night sweats in the lead up to menopause. With disturbed sleep, blood sugar, blood pressure and weight all start to creep up. Studies have shown regular night shifts over extended periods of time can have an adverse effect on health because of disturbed circadian rhythms, increasing the risk of **obesity**, heart attacks, type 2 diabetes, menstrual irregularity and even the risk of breast cancer.[1,2] Insomnia if unresolved in menopause could have similar effects.

Insomnia and sleep apnoea (when breathing stops and starts during sleep) are often underreported in many women with **polycystic ovary syndrome (PCOS)** and can persist through to menopause and may even get worse.

During the perimenopause, pelvic pain and painful periods can disturb sleep, especially if there are underlying conditions such as endometriosis or adenomyosis. Endometriosis can be associated with pain, stress, chronic fatigue, and depression, all of which can affect sleep. In fact, pain of any kind, especially chronic pain, can affect sleep quality.

Disturbed nights lead to further hormonal disruption. This can lead to chronic sleep deprivation, snoring and less restful sleep. This vicious cycle should be addressed early to avoid worsening of symptoms.

Menopause and sleep

Insomnia because of vasomotor symptoms appears to be the most common sleep disorder in women around menopause.

Hot flushes, the most common symptom around menopause, are associated with sleep disturbances. Hot flushes may wake you up, sometimes drenched in sweat (known as night sweats). Once awake, it is harder to go back to sleep and when this happens repeatedly, chronic sleep deprivation sets in. This may be one of the reasons you feel tired in the morning. Dropping oestrogen levels is considered to be an important factor but falling progesterone levels could also contribute to sleep disturbances around the menopause.

Mood changes, anxiety, stress, and depression affect sleep, with many women finding they take longer to fall asleep or notice early morning waking.

Women in the perimenopause who are suffering from hot flushes appear to have a higher chance of being depressed. The years around menopause can be a stressful time for many because of the worry of perhaps caring for elderly parents, personal relationship problems, finances, or children leaving home for jobs, college or university or not leaving at all.

Studies show sleep is disturbed for three to four women in ten in the perimenopause and at least half (50 per cent) suffering in menopause.[3,4] Women who have surgical menopause (removal of functioning ovaries) seem to be at higher risk of sleep problems due to the sudden withdrawal of hormones.

Research shows that peri- and post-menopausal women experience sleep disturbances, even in the absence of hot flushes. There are over 34 symptoms described in menopause and many of them are interlinked with poor sleep, including body weight issues, low libido and urinary frequency.

Other sleep disorders such as sleep apnoea (when your breathing stops and starts while you sleep), restless legs syndrome, or both, are also seen more commonly in menopause.

Urinary frequency can wake you up several times at night, resulting in broken sleep. Cystitis, urinary infections, poorly controlled diabetes, pelvic floor dysfunction, and pelvic organ prolapse can all contribute to urinary urgency and frequency, with a need to pass urine often, sometimes just in small quantities, but enough to wreck one's sleep. Many of these conditions, once recognized, can be managed satisfactorily, with the help of lifestyle advice, physiotherapy, medications or surgery as appropriate.

Helping yourself

If you think you are sleep deprived, are not feeling refreshed after a night's sleep, or if you are constantly tired during the day, try to follow some of the suggestions below. If restful sleep still eludes you, ask to be referred by your family doctor to a sleep clinic or specialist. Sleep issues are best addressed early as disturbed sleep has many unwanted effects, especially if it persists over an extended period of time.

I suggest starting by keeping a detailed diary every day for a week if possible, noting any particular stress, naps, alcohol, caffeine and food intake, as well as logging your exercise regime and your sleep. This will help identify any obvious areas that you can start to address. It could involve any one aspect of your lifestyle, be it exercise, nutrition, stress management or cutting back on alcohol and caffeine as you may find making a small change has a positive effect on your sleep.

Keeping a journal detailing your emotions may also be useful and make for better sleep, so you are not taking your worries to bed.

Morning light is particularly helpful to suppress melatonin and get you ready for the day. Regular physical movement and exercises such as swimming, yoga, dancing, or going to the gym can all help with a good night's sleep, with intense workouts ideally done earlier in the day. Gardening, walking, or spending time in nature can be especially relaxing.

A short nap of less than 30 minutes, not more than an hour, earlier in the day has been shown to be beneficial for health, and can work well for some of you, while meditation and simple mindfulness techniques can reduce your stress levels and improve sleep quality.

Both alcohol and caffeine can act as stimulants and can disturb sleep. They can also increase urinary frequency, often at night. Instead, consider drinking caffeine-free herbal teas, such as chamomile, a couple of hours before bedtime, keeping caffeinated drinks to the early part of the day. Nicotine can also affect your sleep adversely.

The foods you eat and the timings of your meals can make a difference to your sleep quality. Eating your main meal early, ideally before 7 pm, in tune with the circadian rhythm (your body's 'internal clock'), or at least a couple of hours before going to bed, helps with restful sleep by reducing reflux and indigestion. Avoid going to bed hungry or too full.

A complex carbohydrate starch-based protein-rich meal, such as beans or tofu with sweet potatoes, is ideal as it keeps you fuller for longer. A Mediterranean-style plant-predominant diet is associated with adequate sleep duration and fewer insomnia symptoms.

Going to bed the same time every day and sleeping in a darkened cool room, perhaps with an eye mask, can make a difference to the quality of your sleep. Avoid spending waking hours in bed on a regular basis, as your brain stops associating your bed with sleep. Ensuring you are tired and ready for bed will help make you want to go to sleep rather than dreading the night ahead. Consider layers of bedclothes to avoid overheating which can result in a restless night, especially if you are struggling with hot flushes and night sweats. Cooling blankets can be good for night sweats too.

Bright lights, television and smartphones can all suppress melatonin, a hormone produced in the brain, the levels of which need to rise in the evening to enable us to fall asleep. It is a good idea to remove all electronic devices from the bedroom that emit the blue light that suppresses melatonin. Unwind with a pleasant book or soothing music to relax your mind or take a bath. Avoid setting alarms to allow your body to wake up naturally. If you do need one, an old-fashioned alarm clock might be a good option.

Some people will benefit from psychological approaches, of which cognitive behavioural therapy for insomnia (CBT-I) appears to be the most effective treatment. CBT-I has been shown to effectively treat menopause-related insomnia disorder, and has been found to be better than sleep hygiene education alone. Sleeping pills or antidepressants may help some of you, but this should be a carefully considered decision taken on medical advice, and ideally for a short period of time, while exploring other avenues. Lifestyle changes and CBT-I should ideally be tried before sedatives.

Consider a digital wearable which tracks sleep and prompts healthy sleep habits if you need motivation or guidance. There are several on the market but remember, they cannot be completely relied upon without accompanying behaviour change, and they come with a price tag.

Talk to your healthcare professional and make them aware of your sleep issues, even if they do not specifically ask. With the help of detailed questions, your doctor should be able to come to a diagnosis – not all sleep disturbance is menopause related.

Hormone replacement therapy can help with hot flushes and may help improve sleep, but not in everybody, especially if your sleep disturbance isn't related to vasomotor symptoms such as hot flushes or night sweats. A trial of HRT, if appropriate, is certainly worth considering, after a proper informed discussion. Maintaining as many of the changes discussed will hopefully help you sleep better in the long run. Sleep deprivation is real and detrimental to your health, so make it a priority.[5] You might not be able to control all the factors that interfere with your sleep, but you can adopt habits that encourage the restful sleep you deserve.

The importance of sleep

- Getting restful sleep for an adequate amount of time is essential for general wellbeing and hormonal health.
- Insomnia is a common complaint of menopause.
- Insomnia because of hot flushes, night sweats, anxiety or low-level depression is the most common sleep disorder in women around menopause.
- Hormonal fluctuations, stress, sleep apnoea, period pain, chronic pain, restless leg syndrome and urinary problems can affect sleep quality and sleep duration.
- Good quality sleep is needed for cell repair, immunity, memory building, brain and heart health, weight maintenance, stress reduction, improved mood and better relationships.
- Disrupted circadian rhythms from disturbed sleep can increase risk of chronic illness.
- Lifestyle changes and cognitive behaviour therapy for insomnia (CBT-I) should be tried before sedatives.
- Seek specialist help early, especially if you snore or have sleep apnoea issues.

Menopause mantra: *I will not take my worries to bed*

- Find out how much sleep you need to feel rested.
- Start the day with morning light to suppress melatonin.
- Go to bed at the same time each day.
- Have a regular bedtime routine, starting at least an hour before you fall asleep.
- Spend time in nature and exercise regularly.
- Avoid blue light before bedtime.
- Avoid caffeine after midday.
- Eat your dinner at least 2–3 hours before going to bed.
- Avoid alcohol.
- Use your bed for just sleep and sex.
- Keep your bedroom cool and use layers rather than thick quilts.
- Limit daytime naps to 30 minutes, not more than an hour.
- Consider CBT-I for insomnia before medications.
- Consider HRT.
- Seek professional help.

21

Life in the fast lane: The effects of stress

The word 'stress' was not part of my vocabulary growing up in India, where people around me tended to have a fatalistic approach to life. I am sure people were stressed, they just did not have a word for it, probably as most Indians were busy trying to survive by eking out a living on a day-to-day basis. I remember being grateful to have water and electricity at least some days in the week, and feeling happy when the lights came back on. The fast pace of life has overtaken people not just in India but all over the world in the last couple of decades, and most of us will freely admit to being chronically stressed nowadays.

Stress can be acute or chronic. It is the way our body reacts to a real or perceived threat, often making us feel under pressure and out of control.

Acute stress feels intense and occurs quickly, usually within a few hours of an upsetting event, and is short lasting, typically less than a few weeks. Examples include losing a loved one or a breakup or a natural disaster.

Chronic stress on the other hand, as the term implies, either lasts a long time or keeps returning. You might experience this if you feel under pressure a lot of the time, juggling many roles or if your day-to-day life is difficult, for example if you have a chronic health condition, work, financial or relationship concerns.

In our hectic modern-day lives, stress is an invisible factor in most health conditions, with 81 per cent of women in the UK admitting to regularly feeling overwhelmed. Chronic stress puts our health at risk, increasing our risks of chronic illness including heart disease, hypertension, stroke and type 2 diabetes. Weight gain, anxiety, depression, headaches, sleep problems, poor concentration, body aches, digestive problems and hormonal dysregulation can all increase in the presence of chronic stress. While it has many other important functions in our body, cortisol is known as the 'stress' hormone, and it can remain chronically elevated in chronic stress. Adrenaline, the hormone responsible for the fight or flight response, insulin, prolactin, growth and thyroid hormones can also be elevated in chronic stress.[1]

Work-related stress was cited as the reason for feeling unwell by 44.8 per cent of staff in the 2022 NHS survey. Stress, alongside anxiety and other psychiatric illnesses, is consistently the most reported reason for sickness absence in the NHS, accounting for nearly half a million full time equivalent days lost.[2]

Some stress is good for us and can motivate us in some situations, helping us achieve goals we may set ourselves, be it for meeting work deadlines, hosting a dinner party or giving a presentation.

Perimenopause, menopause and stress

Symptoms of stress vary from woman to woman. Feeling irritable, angry, anxious, mood swings, panic attacks, short-term memory loss, lack of concentration and even suffering from severe mental and physical exhaustion are symptoms experienced by women around menopause due to hormonal fluctuations, but these could also be due to chronic stress.

The hormonal fluctuations in perimenopause and early years of menopause can worsen stress and anxiety levels in many women, making the workplace environment particularly challenging (Chapter 21).

Menopause and depression

Women around menopause are at an increased risk of depression and depressive disorders, with feelings of sadness, loss of interest in normal activities, weight loss and irritability, if they have suffered depression when younger, according to the North American Menopause Society.[3] Depression can spike, especially in perimenopause, making women vulnerable to crippling isolation.[4]

As depression is associated with a chemical imbalance in the brain, it is important to seek medical advice if you think you may be depressed, as there are many effective treatments available, from **CBT** or talking therapy to prescription medications, depending on the level of depression. These can help to significantly improve your quality of life. Counselling and therapy should be tried first, as they are safe and proven therapies, alongside medications if they are prescribed.

Helping yourself

How one deals with stress in perimenopause and menopause depends on a large number of factors, including genetics, our upbringing, our life experiences, our support networks and access to treatments.

Stress can affect self-esteem, mood and sleep, all of which can affect our food choices and make us avoid social interactions, exercise and other healthy behaviours and encourage us to turn to alcohol or drugs. When your stress levels are low, consider putting in place strategies to avoid such harmful behaviours and to help you deal with stressful situations better. Figuring out if your stress is acute or chronic or whether most of your symptoms are linked to the hormonal fluctuations of perimenopause and menopause can be useful to get the right treatment, including hormone therapy (see above).

Regular exercise, sleep and breathwork

Physical activity can help you to manage your stress and anxiety levels. Initially you may find it hard to motivate yourself, so try doing something simple like a walk, or a yoga class with a loved one. Spending time outdoors in nature or with companion animals has been found to ease stress. Prioritize sleep, as this can be an issue around menopause and disturbed sleep tends to worsen stress, mood and concentration issues. Learn to focus on your breathing and on slowing it down as it can help when faced with a stressful situation.

Dietary choices

Consciously add more colourful fruit and vegetables into your daily diet as the intake of these anti-inflammatory foods reduces the very hormones that increase our stress levels.

Diets high in refined grains, sweets, red and processed meat and high-fat dairy products have been consistently associated with lower scores of health-related quality of life including mood, compared with plant-predominant diets. Depression can be helped by cutting out ultra-processed foods, as they often contain various compounds and additives that can affect mood. Keep away from alcohol, tobacco and drugs as these will worsen stress and your health, especially in the longer term.

Stress management techniques

Studies have found psychological and behavioural interventions such as mindfulness-based stress reduction (MBSR) interventions can be effective in reducing menopause-related symptoms.[5,6,7] MBSR may also help in reducing the frequency but not the intensity of hot flushes.

Gratitude practices and thinking of any positive aspects that are going well in your life can help relieve stress levels. Yoga, meditation, simple mindfulness and breathing techniques can help calm the mind and reduce anxiety levels. Volunteering in your community, cultivating hobbies that you are interested in or finding groups online that are experiencing perimenopause and menopause are other options to help you manage your stress levels.

Writing your fears or concerns in a diary or journal may help you to see the situation more clearly. By identifying and acknowledging stress triggers, you may feel better equipped to deal with the situation. Talking about your fears with a trusted friend or family member may help you feel better.

Sexual dysfunction, urinary or bowel symptoms, often associated with menopause, can cause stress and embarrassment. There is plenty of help available, so do talk to a health professional.

Finally, if none of these suggestions appeals to you or has been of much use, I would suggest seeking medical advice from a qualified health professional, as therapy such as CBT can make a difference. Some of you may benefit from taking medications. You can still continue with lifestyle modifications alongside this.

Stress

- Stress is the body's reaction to threat and can be acute or chronic.
- Chronic stress increases the risk of chronic illness such as heart disease, hypertension, stroke and type 2 diabetes.
- Other effects of stress include weight gain, mood changes, headaches, sleep problems, poor concentration, body aches and digestive problems.
- Cortisol, adrenaline, thyroid and other hormones are often raised in chronic stress.
- Hormonal fluctuations around menopause can worsen stress.

- Many of the symptoms of menopause are similar to those of stress.
- Women around menopause are at an increased risk of depression and depressive disorders, with a spike around perimenopause.

Menopause mantra: *I will plan ahead to help reduce my stress levels.*

- Identify and acknowledge stress triggers to be able to put strategies in place.
- Regular physical activity and a focus on restful sleep will help reduce stress.
- Eating whole plant foods while reducing ultra-processed foods can help improve mood.
- Spending time in nature, breathwork, keeping a journal, volunteering are known stress relievers.
- Stress management techniques such as gratitude practices, yoga, meditation are helpful.
- Mindfulness-based stress reduction techniques can help reduce stress in menopause.
- CBT, counselling, talking therapy should be considered first for stress management.
- HRT may help in some women and sometimes prescription medications may be needed.
- Seek professional help early.

22

The solution is not in that glass: Risky substance use

It is rather easy to reach for that glass of wine, then another and yet another. Before one knows it, half a bottle of wine or more has been downed, and it soon becomes a regular event on several days of the week. In a society where alcohol is normalized, we convince ourselves that we need that drink to relax because we have had a stressful day at work or because of family matters or just because it's the weekend.

Dealing with anxiety, hot flushes and mood changes, symptoms commonly associated with perimenopause and menopause, whilst also having to manage life events around this time can genuinely be a struggle for many of us. Women all over the world are often the main carer for ageing parents. At the same time, women can have all or some of the demands of a young family, of children leaving home or staying on at home or a job that has now extra responsibilities as one becomes more senior. This may also be a time when women are re-evaluating whether they wish to remain in a relationship that may not have grown in the way they had hoped. Alcohol can quickly become a crutch to lean on.

Around menopause, women may be in a better financial position, with more free time and disposable income, so eating and drinking out with friends becomes a regular event for many. It is easy in these situations to have several large glasses of wine or cocktails, without giving it much thought.

The scientific evidence

As much as we may enjoy a glass of wine, the science is clear that there are no health benefits from drinking alcohol, regardless of what you may have read or heard. Alcohol is the second most abused drug in our society after nicotine. Alcohol is implicated as a causal factor in more than 60 medical conditions, including high blood pressure, depression, liver disease and seven types of cancer, including breast cancer.

The International Agency for Research on Cancer (IARC) is part of the World Health Organization (WHO) that coordinates and conducts both epidemiological and laboratory research into the causes of human cancer. The IARC has labelled alcohol as a class 1 carcinogen (meaning this substance definitely causes cancer in humans). Other class 1 carcinogens are cigarettes, processed meat, and asbestos.

All alcohol has similar harmful effects, meaning wine has not been shown to be any better than spirits in reducing risk of cancer or vice versa. This is because all alcoholic beverages contain ethanol, which increases levels of acetaldehyde as the alcohol is broken down, which in turn causes cellular DNA damage. Even 1–2 alcoholic drinks ($\geq$ 14–28 g/day) appear to be associated with higher risk of some cancers, including breast cancer.

Breast cancer risk

Alcohol consumption has emerged as the strongest and most consistent dietary factor linked with breast cancer. There is no safe limit to alcohol intake, and even small amounts significantly increase our risk of cancers of the breast and ovary.

Breast cancer is the most common cancer in women (30 per cent of all cases), according to Cancer Research UK. One in seven women will receive a diagnosis of breast cancer in their lifetime in the UK. It appears that almost one in four (23 per cent) of breast cancer cases in the UK are preventable, although a person's risk of developing cancer depends on many factors, including age and genetics.

We worry a lot about the risks of breast cancer with the combined oral contraceptive pill (COCP or hormonal birth control pill) and hormone replacement therapy (HRT) but in reality, less than 1 in 100 of breast cancer in the UK is caused by taking long-term COCP oral contraceptives and around 2 in 100 of breast cancer cases in the UK are caused by post-menopausal hormone therapy.

On the other hand, 8 in 100 of breast cancer cases in the UK are caused by alcohol and another 8 per cent by carrying excess weight (overweight and obesity). Cigarette smoking also increases the risk of breast cancer, although this is not widely talked about, with the risk being the highest in women who start smoking in their early teens. Active and passive smoking both increase the risk of breast cancer.

Women who have three alcoholic drinks per week have a 15 per cent higher risk of breast cancer compared to non-drinkers. Even a single small additional drink (100 ml of wine or 10 g of ethanol) each day is estimated to increase the risk of breast cancer by another 9 per cent in post-menopausal women, as per the World Cancer Research Fund and the American Institute for Cancer Research data.

Alcohol and heart health

You may have heard that there could be a protective effect for your heart if you drink red wine regularly. This is not true as previous studies may have failed to account for large numbers of former drinkers and unhealthy individuals with chronic illnesses in the 'non-drinker' category, meaning by default those in the 'drinker' category had healthier lifestyles. Experts are clear that the consumption of alcohol is not simply a trade-off between cancer risk and cardiovascular risk.

Alcohol intake guidelines

In August 2022, Canadian guidelines[1] based on current evidence recommended that men and women should restrict alcohol intake to reduce alcohol-related health risks. The guidance explains there is an incremental risk with having alcohol. Having no drinks per week promotes better health and sleep. If one is going to consume alcohol, then less than two standard drinks a week is best if you wish to avoid alcohol-related health issues. A standard drink or a unit in the UK has 8 g of pure alcohol, which is roughly a small glass of wine, half a pint of beer, lager or cider or an alcopop. In the USA, one standard drink has 14 g of pure alcohol and is equivalent to 1.77 (1¾ unit drinks in the UK). Three to six standard drinks a week increases our risk of cancers, while seven or more drinks increases our risks of heart disease and stroke. Each additional standard drink radically increases the risk of alcohol-related consequences, including injuries and violence.

Alcohol can affect the action of many of the common prescription drugs you may be taking to treat conditions such as raised blood pressure, type 2 diabetes and raised cholesterol, as well as many anxiety medications, sleeping pills, certain antibiotics and antidepressants.

Alcohol in these situations can sometimes have harmful effects, but can also make you feel more tired and impact your reaction times.

Cigarette smoking

Tobacco use is still, unfortunately, the leading preventable cause of cancer and cancer deaths, being implicated in as many as 14 different types of cancer, including cancer of the cervix and ovary, with the toxic chemicals in cigarettes causing DNA and cell damage in various organs and not just the lungs. Smoking significantly worsens the risk of metabolic syndrome, insulin resistance and higher triglyceride levels, which in turn increases the risks of heart disease and stroke in both men and women. Vaping or e-cigarettes are also not as safe as the manufacturers may lead the public to believe. Most clinicians have significant reservations about vaping and rightly so, as there are links to health problems such as addiction, breathing problems, organ damage and even cancer.

Drug misuse

In 2021, a staggering one in five women aged 18 or older reported using illicit drugs (defined as federally illegal drugs, including cannabis, and misuse of prescription medications) in the past 12 months.[2]

Women face unique challenges when it comes to substance use, dose and effects being quite different from those experienced by men, but this is often not taken into consideration. Women say they use drugs for weight reduction, to combat tiredness, pain management and even self-treating mental health issues. Divorce, loss of child custody, or the death of a partner or child can trigger women's substance use, which in turn worsens panic attacks, anxiety and depression.

Effects on menopause

Alcohol and tobacco smoking can have negative effects on mood, hot flushes and sleep, making already existing symptoms of perimenopause and menopause worse. Recent stress, anxiety or depression related to menopause may trigger the onset of alcohol abuse or worsen alcohol habits.

Studies confirm women who misuse drugs can have issues related to all aspects of hormonal health, including menstrual cycle disturbances and menopause.

Tobacco smoking is more likely to bring forward the onset of menopause 18 months earlier for women who smoke compared to those who do not.[3] Passive smokers also seem to be at risk of an earlier menopause. Menopause onset could be up to three or four years earlier for heavy smokers. Nicotine disrupts the conversion of the androgen hormone androstenedione to oestrogen, which results in lower oestrogen levels over time, triggering earlier menopause and worsening menopausal symptoms, especially hot flushes. Smoking negatively affects bone health, worsening osteoporosis risk. Cigarette smoking also hastens premature ageing, affecting hair and skin, an issue already for many women in menopause.

While low to moderate alcohol consumption may be associated with a later onset of menopause and a lower risk of early menopause,[4] this not necessarily a good thing. This is due to the effect alcohol has on raising levels of oestrogen, the mechanism likely involved in increasing hormone receptor positive breast cancer.

Hot flushes and night sweats can be triggered by alcohol intake. Restful sleep, already hard to come by in this phase of life, is worsened by alcohol intake.

Consuming extra calories not just from alcohol but also from poorer food choices made when drinking alcoholic beverages, for example choosing chips instead of a healthier option, can cause unwanted weight gain, already an issue in menopause. Consumption of alcohol, especially beer, appears to be associated with an increased risk of developing fibroids throughout a woman's lifetime.

What's clear from the science is that no matter where you are currently, to improve your health, the less alcohol you drink the better. Stopping smoking is one of the best things you can do for your health and will have immediate positive effects.

Helping yourself

We have established that there are no safe limits for alcohol, cigarettes or illicit drugs and my medical advice is to avoid them as much as possible. However, change can feel overwhelming. I suggest setting yourself small achievable goals. Start with identifying your triggers, perhaps noting them down in a diary over a couple of weeks, helping you to avoid situations in advance that would encourage alcohol, smoking or drug misuse. Reiterate to yourself why you want to make changes, perhaps journal some of those feelings as they will inevitably rise.

Remind yourself that reaching out for support, counselling and therapy can help the journey positively, whether it is through your doctor or various independent organizations. The NHS Quit Smoking app and various helplines may be other ways of supporting you in your decision. Getting friends and family that you trust on board can be helpful, but one needs to be firm as your intentions may get derailed by well-intentioned people who mistakenly think a drink or a cigarette won't hurt your progress.

Consider planning ahead by setting specific alcohol-free days, removing all temptation from your home, or having a set period of abstinence. Smart swaps such as swapping a cigarette for a telephone call with a friend or a warm bath or a healthy snack, or an alcoholic drink for a sparkling water with lemon or non-alcoholic unsweetened beverage, choosing lower alcoholic beverages, taking smaller sips are just some suggestions (see also the resources at the end of the book).

If you choose not to drink, smoke or misuse drugs, you do not need to explain yourself to others. A simple *no* should suffice but you may wish to engage and say you want to look after your health better and that support and encouragement are welcome. If you do feel the urge to indulge, remind yourself that most urges are temporary and will pass. Finding a distraction or keeping busy with a healthy activity at such times may help you. This could be painting, dancing to music or going for a gentle jog or anything you enjoy.

A variety of reasons including societal judgement, cultural presence of alcohol, targeting of women by the alcohol industry means that women can have difficulty in gaining access to treatment and support. This should not put you off, but instead be aware that professional help is available, and you should demand it.

Health professionals have a duty of care to help women reduce their alcohol and drug intake. Studies have repeatedly shown that a doctor advising against alcohol and cigarette smoking has the most power on a patient to make positive changes, as the public still regard a doctor's recommendation as more influential than any other source of information. The use of a screening tool while dispelling pervading myths about the benefits of alcohol can be particularly helpful in identifying women at risk.

Risks of substance use

- There are zero health benefits from drinking alcohol, based on scientific evidence.
- Alcohol is the second most abused drug after nicotine.
- Alcohol is implicated as a causal factor in high blood pressure, depression, liver disease and seven types of cancer.
- As few as three standard alcoholic drinks per week increase the risk of breast cancer significantly.
- 8 in 100 cases of breast cancer are caused by alcohol.
- Alcohol can affect prescription medications.
- Tobacco smoking is the leading preventable cause of cancer and cancer-related deaths.
- Smoking can cause earlier menopause, premature ageing and affects bone health.
- Both smoking and alcohol worsen hot flushes, anxiety and sleep in menopause.
- Alcohol can cause unwanted and unhealthy weight gain.
- One in five women aged 18 or older reported using illicit drugs.
- Professional help through a doctor, helpline or organization can save lives.

Menopause mantra: *I can say no without any further explanations*

- Identify your triggers.
- Keep a diary.
- Plan ahead to avoid environments that encourage the habit you are trying to give up.
- Remind yourself why you want to make the change.
- Speak to a trusted person who will support you.
- Consider counselling or therapy for support.
- Make smart swaps: choose sparkling water or a non-alcoholic drink instead of alcohol.
- Ring a friend or choose a healthy snack instead of the cigarette or drug.
- Remember urges are temporary and will pass.
- Distract yourself with a warm bath, painting, reading, walk with a friend, dancing, cooking or anything you fancy.

23

Menopause mates: Finding that support

The feeling of isolation and not fully knowing where to turn for support during my much earlier than expected menopause is still clear in my mind. It was understandably difficult for my friends and family to fully comprehend the effect my erratic hot flushes, anxiety and lowered libido was having on my mental health, especially as I was not aware of anyone of my age in a similar situation as myself. I did not share as much as I could have about what I was experiencing, not even with my husband Rajiv, as I hadn't really connected the dots until my periods completely stopped, putting most of my symptoms initially down to stress. Like many women, I didn't want to make a fuss; after all, I was not unwell or seriously ill, so what was the point of drawing attention to my 'vague' symptoms? Work and family kept me busy, so I pushed on instead of reaching out which, in hindsight, would have been so much better for me.

This experience of feeling isolated when faced with these symptoms is not limited to but may be felt more intensely by those going through an earlier menopause (POI or early menopause). Hearing friends talk about dating, contraception, fertility and pregnancies when you are dealing with hot flushes and vaginal dryness, especially in your 20s and 30s, can be a real challenge.

My patients in their 50s and 60s mention similar feelings of isolation (often emotional rather than physical), especially when they were transitioning into menopause and still having periods. They remember suffering many of the symptoms of the perimenopause and menopause, such as feeling disproportionately tired, having disturbed sleep, feeling irritable, having little or no sex drive and/or a foggy brain, but did not recognize them as linked to menopause because in reality there has been little awareness raised amongst the public about many aspects of women's health. The perimenopause and menopause are no exceptions.

Human connections

We are social creatures and human relationships are important for our health. The COVID-19 pandemic and the enforced social isolation brought that home very clearly to us, having a severe impact on mood and anxiety in all age groups. Zoom chats helped many people, including myself. I was grateful for our regular Zoom book club meets where we chatted about so much more than the book we had just read, while sharing a drink or meal online.

There appear to be powerful scientific reasons why in-person social functions and gatherings, whether it's attending a lunch with friends, a religious function, or a celebratory occasion, are good for us, influencing our long-term health and longevity just as much as the other five lifestyle pillars we have discussed so far. Pleasant social interactions allow for sharing of knowledge and ideas, as well as being an opportunity for both physical and emotional support. Studies have found social connections can help relieve harmful levels of stress and caring behaviours trigger the release of stress-reducing hormones. It appears that the positive effects of social support extend to the giver as well as the receiver.

One large study of over 300,000 people found that lack of strong relationships increased the risk of premature death from all causes by 50 per cent – an effect on mortality risk roughly comparable to smoking up to 15 cigarettes a day, and greater than obesity and physical inactivity. Relationships can help maintain and improve memory and reduce the risk of depression. By associating with people who have healthy habits, we also seem to benefit by adopting similar behaviours.[1,2]

The Blue Zones

The longevity of the people who live in the five 'Blue Zones' in the world is in part attributed to their interpersonal connections. The Blue Zones are in Nicoya in Costa Rica, Ikaria in Greece, Sardinia in Italy, Loma Linda in California and Okinawa in Japan, where there are a high number of centenarians and very low levels of chronic disease. People tend to follow all six lifestyle pillars diligently as a way of life, and mostly eat a plant-predominant diet (95 per cent whole plant foods).

Studies have shown that those with positive relationships tend to enjoy better health and immunity and even live longer. In contrast, loneliness and isolation are associated with chronic stress and poor health outcomes, especially among individuals already diagnosed with health conditions. According to Age UK, more than 2 million people in England over the age of 75 live alone, and more than 1 million older people say they go for over a month without speaking to a friend, neighbour or family member.

Menopause and social support

There is evidence that having social support helps ease many perimenopausal and menopausal symptoms, including hot flushes, anxiety and even sexual health. This may be in part due to a person feeling seen and heard, which in itself can help improve symptoms.

In a 2022 study, a positive and significant relationship between menopausal symptoms and social support was found, with decreased menopausal symptoms as social support increased.[3] Another 2019 study found greater family support and resilience were significantly associated with fewer menopausal symptoms.[4]

Stress is well documented as worsening vasomotor menopause symptoms. A current stressful event seemed to have the largest effect on menopause symptoms, with 21 per cent more vasomotor symptoms than a woman who had no current stress in a 2021 study.[5]

The changes of perimenopause and menopause can be easier to negotiate when you interact with those who are at a similar stage in their life.[6] Shared experiences tend to make any life event more acceptable, helping lessen that feeling of loneliness.

You may not wish to socialize like you did before and there is no need to. Night clubs, loud music, drinking and eating out may not make you as happy as they might have done in your pre-menopausal years. There are plenty of ways of connecting with others in areas that interest you and may actually be better for your mental and physical health. It is important though that you do it on your terms without having to always explain yourself if you don't feel up to a social engagement.

Depression, relationship issues, panic attacks and difficulties at work with concentration as well as bowel and bladder incontinence can all contribute to women feeling isolated in the perimenopause, often reluctant to leave their home. If you experience these issues, do reach out for professional help.

Women that I speak to are glad there is now a conversation starting around menopause, but many of my older patients say they wish they had had that discussion and support when they were experiencing symptoms and felt isolated and alone. A lot of work still remains to be done in the USA and the UK and around the world to improve understanding about the perimenopause and menopause.

Helping yourself

Who can blame women for wanting to withdraw from social interactions when so many unfathomable changes are occurring in one's body? Without the knowledge of the workings of the female reproductive organs, hormones and the different phases that women experience in their lifetime, menopause can feel overwhelming.

I want you to be in control, using the knowledge that you have gathered from reliable resources to get appropriate help rather than feeling vulnerable and at a loss. It is usually the unknown that worries most people, making them fearful.

I encourage you to actively start building a meaningful social network of friends who genuinely matter to you and care about you. Reach out to friends or family members who make you feel good about yourself and encourage you.

It is not uncommon to feel anxious, underconfident about your appearance or have physical symptoms such as bladder urgency, sweating or flushing, all of which may make you feel more reluctant to socialize, but help is available for most of these symptoms. It is important to be able to advocate for oneself to be heard.

Whether your isolation is self-imposed or involuntary, studies have shown it is better for your health to have social interactions on a regular basis. Many chronic illnesses including dementia, depression and heart disease are made worse in the presence of loneliness. Being alone is not the same as loneliness and can actually be good for you, particularly at this stage in your life, giving you the time for yourself to do things that you may not have been able to in the past. A good time to draw up a bucket list if that is something that focuses your mind.

Micro interactions also seem to matter in improving mood and wellbeing,[7] so do make it a point to say hello, smile and even have a little chat to people you come across in your day, whether it is on your walk, way to work or at the supermarket. This does not come as easily to me as it does to some of my friends, but I got so much better once I realized it does make me feel so much better. It is also free.

This is a time to prioritize your needs, so surround yourself with people who generally have a positive outlook, helping lift your spirits. Focus on the quality of your relationships rather than the quantity and those who accept you for who you are. The emotional support that you may be looking for may be found, for example, in a local dance, art or walking group, book club, animal shelter volunteer group, with your friends, family members or partner. It can also most definitely be an online group with likeminded people sharing similar experiences and their tips of dealing with their menopause. Getting a rescue dog if you would like the company of an animal at home is also a great way of meeting people and getting exercise at the same time.

Seeking professional help from a therapist, physiotherapist or doctor to address some of your symptoms may be an option for some of you who are struggling to find a way forward or do not find the above suggestions particularly helpful.

Menopause mates: Finding that support

- Feelings of isolation are real in perimenopause and menopause.
- Human connections are important for human health.
- Social interactions improve longevity.
- Interpersonal relations reduce the risk of chronic illnesses including dementia, depression, stress and heart disease.
- Lack of strong relationships increases the risk of premature death from all causes by 50 per cent – similar to smoking up to 15 cigarettes a day, and greater than obesity and physical inactivity.
- Loneliness worsens perimenopausal symptoms.
- Social support helps ease many perimenopausal and menopausal symptoms, including hot flushes, anxiety and even sexual health.
- Positive effects of social support benefit both giver and receiver.
- Relationships can help maintain and improve memory.
- Community can be found in local groups, charities, faith centres.

Menopause mantra: *I will choose my community carefully to find the support I need*

- Reach out to friends and family that encourage healthy behaviours.
- Access appropriate help from qualified professionals.
- Help for menopausal symptoms including anxiety, depression, loneliness is available.
- Local communities and activities such as walking groups or book clubs, or volunteering can be ways to find that emotional support.
- Find online groups of interest to help you through menopause.
- Build positive social connections and surround yourself with people who lift you up.

PART THREE
MY MENOPAUSE

Answering your questions

Over the last three decades, I have had the privilege of looking after hundreds of women in perimenopause, menopause, and in the late post-menopausal phase of their lives, not to mention women to whom I had to break the news of a diagnosis of menopause much earlier than they ever imagined receiving it (see Chapter 1).

Many of the questions my patients ask me have been answered throughout the book, but I have selected a few that come up quite often. Questions on hot flushes, bone health, weight gain, contraception, protein, safety of soya have entire chapters or sections dedicated to the topic. There is a chapter answering the common questions asked about hormone replacement therapy (HRT), although I do address a couple more here. Throughout the book I have used composite case studies to protect the identity of my patients.

I thought this was normal: Period problems

Case: Anna, a 47-year-old Polish interpreter, was seeing me as she had been bleeding continuously for six weeks, with the flow slowing down for a few days and becoming heavy again. She had noticed her periods had become heavier and more painful over the last couple of years, but she had been putting up with it as she thought she was close to menopause. She had two healthy children, both born by emergency caesarean section. She was up to date with her cervical smear but otherwise had never really needed to see a doctor for gynaecological issues.

Perimenopause is often associated with an initial shortening of menstrual cycles, with periods getting more crowded and coming more frequently. As one gets closer to the last menstrual period, women may notice periods skipping some months altogether. This is not always the case.

Heavy or painful periods at any age, including in perimenopause, are not normal

Your periods should come at 25–35-day intervals and bleeding can be anywhere from 1–7 days. If your periods fall out of these ranges, especially for more than three months, or you are worried, you must seek medical advice. Pain that affects your daily life or bleeding that needs double protection (pad plus tampon for example), leaking, flooding or clots larger than your thumb nail (10 pence coin or an American quarter) are not acceptable. Bleeding after sex, prolonged bleeding like in Anna's case or missing periods for months at a time all need a doctor's attention.

A detailed medical history, and pelvic examination if appropriate, along with a pelvic ultrasound scan and blood tests to check for iron-deficiency anaemia can help reach a diagnosis in most women.

Conditions such as fibroids, inflammatory conditions such as endometriosis and adenomyosis, uterine or cervical polyps, PCOS and sometimes cancers of the cervix or uterus can cause prolonged or heavy or irregular periods. PCOS can also be associated with missed periods as can calorie restriction or exercising too much (functional hypothalamic amenorrhoea). All these conditions can persist through perimenopause and need appropriate investigations and medical treatment.

Menopause and gynaecological conditions

My website (www.nitubajekal.com) has detailed information on all these conditions.

PCOS

I discuss the impact of PCOS and menopause in an entire chapter in our book *Living PCOS Free*. Women with PCOS may notice a delay in menopause by about two years. Signs of androgen excess may persist into menopause, with increased hair growth and risks of high blood pressure, abnormal sugar control and higher lipids than other women.

Endometriosis

This is an oestrogen-dependent chronic inflammatory condition where tissue similar to the lining of the uterus sticks itself to various organs, including the bowel, ovaries, bladder and uterus, causing painful heavy periods, chronic fatigue, chronic pelvic pain, painful sex and scar tissue that can affect bladder and bowel function.

Even when periods stop, the effects of the scar tissue (adhesions) in some women can continue to cause pain. Symptoms may flare up with HRT and even after a hysterectomy, combined HRT to quieten the deposits of endometriosis may be needed for a while.

Fibroids

These smooth muscle growths are almost always benign in nature and are very common. While they often cause no issues, fibroids can cause large swellings, heavy periods or irregular bleeding (especially when fibroids protrude into the uterine cavity), as well as bladder and bowel pressure symptoms.

Fibroids tend to shrink in menopause as they are oestrogen-dependent growths, but very large fibroids may still require medical or surgical treatment in perimenopause and menopause. They can sometimes grow in size with HRT, although in general this is not a significant problem.

Adenomyosis

This is also an oestrogen-dependent chronic inflammatory condition and may co-exist with endometriosis, fibroids, and other oestrogen-dependent conditions. In adenomyosis, some of the endometrial lining that sheds every month burrows itself deep into the muscle wall (myometrium) of the womb and continues to grow and bleed each month, enlarging the womb.

Adenomyosis is not a life-threatening condition nor is it cancerous but it can impair quality of life significantly. Painful and/or heavy periods, especially recent onset, chronic pelvic pain, painful sex, fatigue and low iron stores from heavy periods, are commonly seen in this condition. A bulky enlarged uterus which is quite tender on internal examination can be a clue. It may be found as a focus of adenomyosis (known as an adenomyoma) or as generalized adenomyosis on a pelvic MRI scan and sometimes on a pelvic ultrasound scan. Some of the risk factors for adenomyosis include caesarean sections and increasing age.

The condition tends to settle in menopause when hormone levels, especially oestrogen levels, drop and may sometimes flare up again on menopausal hormone therapy.

Medical treatment with hormones or definitive surgery is usually indicated for endometriosis, adenomyosis and symptomatic fibroids, alongside a focus on adding more whole plant foods to one's diet to reduce inflammation, and lifestyle advice.

Case outcome: Anna's symptoms were due to adenomyosis and a large uterine polyp. She responded well to surgical removal of the benign polyp and a progesterone-containing intra uterine system to manage her periods. She wholeheartedly adopted a whole-food plant-based lifestyle and has been doing rather well over the last three years, avoiding further medical interventions.

I don't feel like having sex: Testosterone and low libido

Case: Diane, a 52-year-old accountant, had been on combined HRT for two years but remained unhappy about her lower than previous libido. She had come to see me as she was wondering about testosterone treatment.

Routine use of testosterone as part of HRT is not recommended. While testosterone in the doses recommended for women appears to be safe, long-term studies regarding benefits and safety profile are not available. Testosterone levels plateau in menopause. In my experience, it is sensible to wait six months or so to allow regular HRT to settle in, before considering testosterone. Most women won't need it. Younger women and those with surgical menopause may find it more beneficial, due to sudden drops in level after surgery.

The British Menopause Society (BMS) and the NICE UK guidelines recommend that testosterone is used for low libido after other options have been exhausted, recommending a biopsychosocial approach for women with **hypoactive sexual desire disorder.**[1]

Before prescribing testosterone, I take a detailed history, including details of a woman's physical symptoms of vaginal discomfort or pain during intercourse, which usually responds very well to local measures and additional local vaginal oestrogen which is safe. It is worth asking about the current relationship, and checking if the woman's wishes are realistic.

Some women who are already on HRT with no other psychosexual concerns can benefit with improved sexual function and libido on addition of testosterone. Some women say they find benefits in concentration, mood, energy levels and improved musculoskeletal health, although large-scale studies are not available to confirm this.

Testosterone is prescribed off-licence in the UK, although the preparations prescribed have been used in men for years. Side effects are uncommon with the recommended dosage of 5 mg per day. A menopause-specific 1 per cent testosterone cream is licensed in Australia. Women should not exceed the prescribed dose, as there can be irreversible effects with higher doses (male pattern balding, change in voice, increased size of clitoris).

A baseline blood test for total testosterone levels and a check in 12 weeks can be a helpful guide. However, doses more than 5 mg per day should not be prescribed, and if a woman does not find benefit after six months, testosterone should be discontinued. If she finds it helpful, on annual review of all HRT, a blood test check of the total testosterone level is recommended.[2]

Case outcome: Diane used testosterone for six months but did not find it helped her particularly, despite levels of testosterone rising to the top of the normal range. She decided to continue with her body-identical medically approved HRT gel and tablet and vaginal oestrogen. She stopped the testosterone, but was pleased she had tried it.

Painful sex and bathroom breaks: Genitourinary syndrome of menopause

Case: I had seen Mary, a 62-year-old medical secretary, about 20 years ago to treat her heavy periods, having delivered both her children. I remembered her well. She told me shyly she had met someone special but hadn't taken things forward. She had found sex painful in the last few years of her marriage but had never admitted it, not even to her husband. Now, because of worsening vaginal dryness and soreness, she was apprehensive and felt embarrassed to discuss it with her younger partner. Mary became menopausal at the age of 50. She had tried HRT for a short while, but decided not to continue with it when her husband was diagnosed with cancer. She had lost her husband about five years ago and she had not been sexually active for several years.

It hurts but I can't admit it

Women can suffer from vaginal dryness, soreness, itching and pain at all ages and stages of their lives. We need to talk about painful sex openly, bringing partners into the conversation, so we can raise awareness about the help available, as all women have a right to enjoy sex. A woman may not even realize how much her self-esteem and confidence levels take a knock because of the pain and discomfort she experiences during sex. A feeling of social isolation is very real for many of my patients.

Most women rarely bring up the issue of painful sex during a medical consultation, unless doctors specifically ask them. Women may feel hesitant, thinking they are the only one suffering, especially when one sees everyone in movies and on television enjoying sex at all ages. Women tell me they have put up with it for years, thinking that they will not be taken seriously by their doctor. My patients also say that they did not want to bother their doctor, as there were more important matters for the healthcare system to be dealing with. Painful sex is probably not even a real condition so why make a fuss?

Painful sex

Menopause amplifies the issue of painful sex for many. During menopause, symptoms such as dryness, soreness, pain, burning, irritation, often with no trigger, are usually related to thinning of the lining of the vagina medically known as vaginal atrophy, a term that both my patients and I dislike intensely.

Women often say they feel bruised, describing a sensation of paper cuts and traces of blood after vaginal intercourse. There are oestrogen receptors everywhere, including your bladder and vagina. Falling levels of the hormone oestrogen is the cause for these symptoms in most situations, as one of this hormone's functions is to keep the vaginal tissue lubricated, elastic and supple.

There are physical changes too, with some shrinking of the outer and inner lips, pale or reddened vulval and vaginal skin, blood blisters and reduction in secretions. The acidic vaginal environment changes to a more alkaline one in the menopause, with an increased susceptibility to vaginal and bladder infections.

Genitourinary syndrome of menopause (GSM)

GSM is the term now used to describe symptoms related to oestrogen deficiency, with changes that can involve the labia, introitus, clitoris, vagina, urethra, and bladder. Typically, women notice these symptoms four to six years after their periods completely stop, when the oestrogen reaches very low levels in all tissues. Previous medical terms included atrophic vaginitis, urogenital atrophy, or vulvovaginal atrophy.

Bathroom breaks

Bladder symptoms are part of GSM. Cystitis, in the absence of infection, is a particular problem in menopause, with women needing to pass urine frequently and often with urgency, often passing small amounts. Once again, the lack of oestrogen is usually responsible for this. Women are also more prone to recurrent urinary tract infections (UTIs) in menopause, as the lining of the bladder becomes thin due to a drop in oestrogen, allowing bugs to enter more easily. It is advisable to request a urine test to confirm a UTI before taking unnecessary antibiotics. Blood in your urine should never be ignored.

Vaginal dryness

In older women, this vaginal discomfort and pain combined with a lower libido, often accompanied by disturbed sleep, stress or anxiety all seen more commonly in menopause, can make having sex a chore rather than a pleasure. Younger women, including those in perimenopause, can also be troubled by vaginal dryness. Between 17 and 45 per cent of women in menopause say they find sex painful because of vaginal dryness.[3] Many of them still want to have sex with their partner, but are in pain for days after. As a result, most women either give up on sex, never seeking medical help, or remain silent.

With a combination of natural measures and CBT alongside safe and highly effective medical therapy, many women should be able to enjoy having sex again, should they wish to.

Other causes of painful sex and vaginal soreness

Dyspareunia is the medical term doctors use for painful sex and this can be superficial (on entry) or deep pain. There are many causes of painful sex including vulvodynia and endometriosis, not just menopausal vaginal dryness, so your doctor does need to spend some time getting a thorough medical history and examination to reach a diagnosis and offer you the appropriate treatment. I will not go into greater detail for each individual condition here, but my website has several free fact sheets that may help you (www.nitubajekal.com).

Infections such as thrush and sexually transmitted infections (see Chapter 8) in perimenopause and menopause can cause significant discomfort during sex, but tend to settle with the correct treatment.

Some skin conditions such as eczema, psoriasis, and lichen sclerosus affect the skin of the inner or outer lips of the vulva and can make vaginal symptoms worse.

Autoimmune conditions such as lichen planus can also affect the vagina. Radiotherapy to the female genital organs as part of treatment for cancer can also cause vaginal dryness. There is help available for each of these situations.

Helping yourself

The regular use of water-based vaginal moisturizers, usually two to three times a week, can help keep the vagina moist. Using water-based lubricants before sex makes sexual intercourse more comfortable and should be the first thing you try to manage vaginal dryness, especially in mild cases. It is worth trying different preparations until you find a suitable one. If you have sensitive skin, do check the products carefully as rarely you may be allergic to one or more ingredients.

Caring for your vulva and vagina

There are a few general principles of caring for your vulva and vagina that apply to all ages and whatever the underlying condition. These include avoiding excessive washing, douching, perfumed toiletries, feminine wipes, and toilet wipes, all of which can lead to increased dryness by removing natural body oils and beneficial bacteria, especially in the menopause and for those with sensitive skin. Do not be fooled by products that market themselves as sensitive or kind to the skin, as many products have harsh chemicals that do your skin no favours. Allergies and hypersensitivity to chemicals used in and around the female genital area can cause a great deal of discomfort and soreness.

Think of your vagina as a self-cleansing oven

Consider using just water or a non-soap-based wash in the genital area, but not in excess as this can dry the skin out. The use of natural oils can be beneficial for many women, with the daily application and massage of a small amount of natural oil such as coconut, Vitamin E or almond oil after a shower to lock moisture into the skin in the vulval area, making the area more supple and less irritable.

Using eco-friendly, non-biological laundry detergents which are low in harsh chemicals and using skin-sensitive menstrual incontinence products can all help in relieving vulval and vaginal irritation. Developing sensitivity to laundry detergents and menstrual products is not uncommon.

Go knicker free when you can, especially at night, to air the genital area, as increased heat, moisture, and chafing are perfect settings for infections to take hold. I also suggest changing out of sweaty gym clothes and swimsuits and washing off sweat and chlorine as soon as you can as this may worsen vaginal soreness and discomfort. Breathable cotton over synthetic underwear can help reduce discomfort.

Long courses of antibiotics can strip the vulval and vaginal barrier of healthy bacteria, so one needs to be doubly strict about vulval and vaginal hygiene in such situations.

Eating whole plant foods such as beans, especially soya, fruits such as watermelon and vegetables, can help in improving vaginal lubrication and in improving the vaginal microbiome, aiding the growth of good bacteria.

A stressful lifestyle can also have a significant impact on the quality of sexual health, as can previous sexual experiences, abuse and even encounters with healthcare professionals. Addressing these issues can take time and effort, but things can significantly improve.

Internal examinations can be uncomfortable in menopause, so do warn your doctor and request a smaller lubricated plastic speculum before a smear or vaginal swab test as this can help ease the process.

Regular vaginal intercourse helps to maintain vaginal health and lessen pain over time. My advice, however, is to only have sex if you want to and not because you have to.

Treating GSM with oestrogen

If the moisturizers and lubricants haven't had the effect you were hoping for, be reassured that symptoms of vaginal thinning and dryness respond extremely well to regular use of local vaginal oestrogen. Topical or local vaginal oestrogen comes in the form of a cream, pessary, or vaginal ring containing oestrogen (usually oestradiol or oestriol). This works even better than formal HRT when specifically used for GSM, including treating cystitis because of low oestrogen. After an initial two-week once-a-day application, the cream or pessary is used twice weekly and in some situations, three times a week.

I prefer the use of the cream as some of the cream may be applied to particular sore areas on the vulva or in situations where the applicator can't be used. A vaginal oestrogen ring is changed every three months. All these have similar benefits and it usually comes down to a matter of preference.

Systemic hormone therapy can help with vaginal symptoms on its own but local vaginal treatment can be used alongside formal HRT safely. The oestrogen helps to strengthen the vaginal and bladder lining by improving the blood supply, reducing shedding of cells, and making the thinning tissues plumper and more robust, with improvements noticeable in four weeks for many women. Uncommonly, some women may complain of vaginal irritation, increased discharge, or breast tenderness with local treatment. It will usually settle in a few weeks, but it is helpful to check in with your doctor, especially if you notice any bleeding.

Women can now buy vaginal oestrogen over the counter if they are over the age of 50, with no periods or bleeding for over a year, after a checklist is completed with the pharmacist.

Local low-dose vaginal oestrogen is completely safe for most women and can be used indefinitely, significantly improving quality of life.

It does not raise hormone levels of the oestrogen significantly in the rest of your body. Overgrowth of the lining of the womb (endometrial hyperplasia) is not really a concern at such low doses, even with long-term use, both from studies and in my experience. There has been no increased risk of breast or endometrial cancer, heart disease, clots, or stroke noted with the use of local vaginal oestrogen. It is approved by all expert groups. Even with a history of cancer, including oestrogen-sensitive breast cancer, some experts are comfortable prescribing local vaginal oestrogen, but individualized discussions with your oncology team are important if there is any doubt. Your partner also does not need to worry about absorption of oestrogen.

The use of reusable graduated silicone vaginal dilators that gently stretch the vagina, along with all the measures described, may be of help to some women. These are easily available online and are not particularly expensive. The advantage with dilators is that you can do this in your own time, as often as you wish to, and in private. It has been instrumental in helping my patients achieve successful intercourse in combination with vaginal oestrogen.

Pelvic floor physiotherapy and working with a trusted professional can also be extremely beneficial.

There are some other newer treatments that may be considered on an individualized basis (local selective oestrogen receptor modulators, known as SERMs have minimal or no effect on other oestrogen-sensitive tissues such as the breast, while benefiting the vagina), vaginal dehydroepiandrosterone DHEA suppositories, vaginal testosterone, oral ospemifene for vaginal changes related to menopause, especially when local hormones cannot be used or have failed. We do not have enough evidence yet to recommend routine use of these medications. My advice is that it is best to have an individual consultation with a specialist.

Laser treatment to improve the blood supply and restore collagen and elasticity and moisture in the vaginal tissue may help with painful sex, and may be considered in those women who cannot use oestrogen or if oestrogen has not proved as helpful as hoped. Long-term studies for safety and efficacy for these newer treatments, including radiofrequency and other energy-based therapies, are not available, and therefore they cannot be routinely recommended.

Menopause-related vaginal changes may be an inevitable part of the ageing process but as you can see, there is plenty of help available to manage this very successfully.

Case outcome: After a detailed consultation with Mary and a gentle pelvic examination, I was able to confirm the diagnosis of GSM. Mary was beaming when she sat down about 12 weeks later. She had followed all my instructions for self-care and found the natural oils, local vaginal oestrogen cream and daily use of the vaginal dilators so helpful that she had not only had penetrative vaginal intercourse but had also found it enjoyable. She knew to continue following this advice to the extent she felt comfortable and to seek medical help if she had any future concerns. I discharged a very happy patient.

Menopause mantra: *I will speak up for myself in the doctor's room*

Looking after your vagina:

- Regular use of water-based vaginal moisturizers and lubricants is the first line of treatment.
- Local vaginal oestrogen is safe and highly effective for vaginal atrophy (GSM) for most women.
- Avoid excessive washing, douching, using harsh chemical-laden wipes and perfumed toiletries.
- Use plain water or non-soap-based washes in the genital area.
- Consider application of natural oils such as coconut or vitamin E.
- Switch to skin sensitive laundry and incontinence products.
- Consuming whole plant foods (e.g. soya, watermelon) can help improve vaginal lubrication.
- Breast cancer is not always a contraindication for local vaginal oestrogen therapy.
- There are other treatment options if oestrogen is not suitable.
- Graduated vaginal dilators may help when used regularly.
- There may be other causes of painful sex.
- Request a small plastic lubricated speculum at examination to reduce discomfort.
- Encourage partners to join the discussion.

Don't be fooled: Custom compounded bioidentical HRT

Case: Liz, a 48-year-old home-maker, sat in front of me looking visibly upset. Over the last two years, she had spent thousands of pounds in a private clinic on natural HRT, better known as custom compounded **bioidentical hormones**, on hormone assays, and on many expensive supplements. She mistakenly thought this was safer and better for her than NHS prescribed standard HRT. Despite increasing doses, she had not found much symptom relief. She had gone to see her family doctor for a discussion. When the doctor was not able to fully reassure Liz about the dangers of unregulated hormone therapy and the safety of medically approved HRT, the doctor suggested seeing me for a discussion.

The difference between regulated body identical HRT and bioidentical hormones

Liz is not alone in this misconception that 'natural' equals better. Many women come to me with side effects of vaginal bleeding or medications not working or after realizing they have been spending large sums of money on bioidentical hormones marketed as natural and specifically for them, often accompanied by expensive unproven regular blood, saliva and urinary assays.

Bioidentical hormones are not recommended by any of the Royal Colleges worldwide or by expert groups, as there is no evidence for their safety or efficacy, when compared with standardized HRT.

These custom-compounded, multi-hormone regimens with dose adjustments based upon serial hormone monitoring are not regulated. The doses are not standardized and often deliver large amounts of unopposed hormones or completely ineffective doses, often using unproven routes of administration. As a result, women see variable results, some of them harmful.

While the claim is that bioidentical hormones are natural because they are derived from soya and plant extracts, modified to be structurally identical to our own endogenous hormones, this is also the same approach used for most approved and commercially available regulated modern HRT. The difference is that bioidentical HRT does not come with a safety or efficacy profile.

You may have heard of 'natural' progesterone creams for your skin, along with other dubious bioidentical hormones found online or in physical clinics that have mushroomed all over the world. I would also not recommend these creams as they are not well absorbed into the body to be actually effective. This can be a serious issue as without the right level of progesterone to protect the uterine endometrial lining from unopposed oestrogen, the risks of **endometrial hyperplasia** and cancer are significantly increased.

My advice is to choose standardized **body identical hormones** (the term used to differentiate regulated HRT from unregulated bioidentical hormones) or any of HRT preparations approved by experts and the regulatory bodies, as these have been researched extensively and are carefully monitored. You want to know that any medication you put in or on your body has been through a rigorous safety process. This is the sort of HRT doctors have been prescribing now for a while in the form of gels, patches, pumps, and oral tablets. You might be pleased to hear that horse's urine is no longer used.

Case outcome: After a detailed discussion with Liz, I recommended she switched to effective and regulated HRT. We talked about the importance of lifestyle modifications. She left with resources and happy in the knowledge that she could now approach her doctor for safer HRT medication at a fraction of the cost, especially with the HRT prepayment certificate from the NHS. She realized that choosing quality controlled and medically approved HRT was in her best interest, without the need for unproven and expensive bioidentical hormones or unnecessary hormone tests.

Do I still need it? Cervical screening

Case: Michelle, a 58-year-old sales manager, was seeing me for an unrelated problem. On questioning, she admitted she had been ignoring her cervical screening invitations from the NHS. She had not been sexually active for a while. She was apprehensive of pain and also did not think she was at risk of cervical cancer.

Michelle does need to keep her cervical smear (Pap smear) appointments. Sadly, many women of all ages and backgrounds don't attend the simple screening that can save lives. The reasons are varied and may include fear or pain of the examination as in Michelle's case, concern over the possible results and lack of information and widespread misinformation.

Cervical cancer is the second most common cause of cancer in women all over the world. The good news is that cervical cancer is almost completely preventable. It is caused by the **Human Papilloma Virus** (HPV) infection (99.8 per cent). Certain strains of HPV (Types 16 and 18) are responsible for 70 per cent of all cervical cancers and can be picked up by a simple test. Abnormal cells can be picked up and treated long before cells become cancerous, saving lives. Smoking increases the risk of cervical cancer, so do seek professional support to quit.

Don't miss your smear test as it can save your life

If you have ever been sexually active, then you should attend the NHS cervical screening programme if you live in the UK. Most countries will have a standard screening protocol, which may vary slightly. The NHS offers primary HPV testing between the ages of 25–64 years. After the age of 50, most women need a smear test every five years until the age of 64, unless there is a medical reason to do them more frequently. Self-testing for HPV is being trialled and will be helpful in increasing numbers of women who are screened.

Case outcome: Michelle used a low-dose vaginal oestrogen cream for a couple of weeks to ease the discomfort of vaginal dryness. I talked her through the process and used a small plastic speculum to take the smear, in the presence of a nurse. Michelle was comfortable during the test. She was delighted that her smear was reported clear. She continued with the oestrogen cream as she found it helpful. Read more about HPV and about STIs (sexually transmitted infections) in Chapter 8.

Dropping down: Pelvic organ prolapse

Case: Alison, a 66-year-old grandmother, complained of a dragging sensation and a lump between her legs, especially after a long day looking after her two-year-old grandson. This seemed to have got worse in the last year, affecting her lower back and an incomplete emptying of her bladder, needing to go again as soon as she thought she had finished. She was quite fed up with her symptoms.

Pelvic organ **prolapse**, often simply known as vaginal prolapse or utero vaginal prolapse, is common, affecting one in ten women over the age of 50. This is a condition when the ligaments in the pelvis that normally hold up the internal female organs become relaxed. It is in fact a type of hernia. As a result, one or more of the pelvic organs (cervix, uterus, vagina) drop from their normal position, often dragging the surrounding organs such as the bladder and bowel to create a bulge in the vagina. There are several types of uterovaginal prolapse. Even after surgery for prolapse, the top of the vagina can drop in one to two women in 100, known as a vault prolapse.

A prolapse is not a life-threatening condition but can affect quality of life in some women like Alison, while others do not find it an issue, especially if it is mild. Some women are more prone to developing a prolapse (white women, pregnancy, prolonged childbirth, big babies, genetics, excess body weight, chronic cough, connective tissue diseases etc.). The underlying reasons in individual situations are often hard to define and there can be more than one reason.

Symptoms depend on the kind of prolapse, and include feeling of a vaginal lump, lower back ache, bladder and bowel symptoms. Most prolapse remains the same but may get worse over time, especially with increasing body weight putting excess pressure on the pelvic organs and with oestrogen deficiency in menopause, weakening the ligaments further.

A detailed medical history and thorough internal examination is usually enough to diagnose a prolapse correctly. For those with mild symptoms and even for those who need further treatment, core strength exercises such as Pilates, yoga or pelvic floor physiotherapy and weight loss if needed, can be helpful. Avoiding constipation, smoking and heavy lifting is advised as these can worsen prolapse symptoms. Local vaginal oestrogen can help improve vaginal blood supply and improve the skin texture, reducing discomfort.

Some women opt for a latex or silicone vaginal ring or shelf pessary, especially if they are older, wish to avoid surgery or have multiple medical conditions.

Others will need a surgical procedure, depending on the type of prolapse, general health and the wishes of the woman.

The different surgical options include a number of techniques, either on their own or in combination. The aim is to lift and support the vagina or uterus and cervix and neighbouring organs. Incontinence surgery may be indicated and offered at the same time. Operations include pelvic floor repair, surgery for a vault prolapse and even a hysterectomy (removal of uterus and cervix). If you wish for more detailed information, please refer to the fact sheets on my website (www.nitubajekal.com).

Case outcome: After a thorough assessment and discussion, Alison opted for a surgical procedure. She was not keen on waiting or to try a pessary. I agreed with her. I prescribed local vaginal oestrogen cream to help strengthen the tissues for a few weeks in the lead up to surgery and indefinitely post-surgery as well as following a healthy diet to improve recovery. I performed a keyhole hysterectomy with removal of her uterus, cervix, fallopian tubes and ovaries along with a pelvic floor repair. She remains delighted with her decision more than five years later.

Don't ignore that spotting: Post-menopausal bleeding (PMB)

Case: Linda, a 61-year-old retired teacher, noticed spotting out of the blue on wiping herself. It lasted for a few days. She was otherwise well in herself with no medical concerns and was not on HRT. She knew to seek medical advice urgently.

Post-menopausal bleeding

Any vaginal bleeding after the menopause (12 months of no periods) is known as post-menopausal bleeding (PMB) and should be taken seriously.

Most women who have PMB do not have cancer, but it is the most serious cause of PMB. Uterine cancer, the most common cancer of the female genital tract in the UK, when picked up early has a good prognosis.

There are many benign and more common reasons why women have PMB. These include thinning of the vagina and uterine lining because of low levels of oestrogen in menopause, HRT use, uterine or cervical polyps (grape-like growths from the lining), fibroids and vulval skin conditions such as blood blisters and lichen sclerosus. Other less common causes could be bleeding from the urinary tract or bowel, certain drugs such as blood thinning agents and vaginal infections. Treatment depends on the cause.

PMB can be a sign of cancer of the cervix, uterus or vagina, with approximately one in ten of women with PMB having uterine cancer. The incidence increases with increasing age.

Women are advised to have tests, such as a pelvic scan, blood tests and a sample of the lining of the womb, depending upon the medical history and a physical examination. These investigations are done to check there is no underlying reason for the bleeding such as endometrial (womb) cancer. Women in the UK are often referred to the hospital as a two-week urgent referral, so that they can be seen quickly and reassured.

Case outcome: Linda had a transvaginal pelvic ultrasound which confirmed a thin endometrial lining, putting her at negligible risk of cancer. She was up to date with her cervical smear. The cause in her case was menopause-related thinning of the vagina and I prescribed her local vaginal oestrogen to help improve the vaginal tissue and reduce the risk of further episodes. She would continue to see her GP and I explained I was happy for her to continue with the oestrogen cream for the foreseeable future if it was helping her. I also suggested some other vulval and vaginal measures. I reassured her and discharged her back to her doctor. She knew to seek medical advice if she had bleeding in the future or any other health concerns.

PART FOUR
MENOPAUSE MORSELS

Menopause-friendly recipes (with health tips)

I am excited to share some of my favourite recipes with you here. I focus on beans, lentils and soya in my recipes as these nutritious foods are particularly menopause friendly. These flavoursome dishes contain protein, fibre, complex carbohydrates, are naturally low in saturated fat, full of micronutrients and easy to prepare.

Most of my recipes are oil and gluten-free but can be adapted to suit any diet.

I'll be sharing what a typical day of meals could look like, but this is by no means prescriptive. You can also easily adapt the recipes to suit your palate.

I also share three recipes from The Happy Menopause Course that I co-host with The Happy Pear,[1] David and Steven Flynn, brilliant cooks, friends and menopause allies. Dr Rajiv and Rohini each share one of their favourite recipes, as does my dear friend Daisy Koizia. I hope you and your loved ones will enjoy these dishes as much as we do and that in time they find a regular place on your dining table.

A typical menopause menu

Breakfast – I recommend porridge/oatmeal regularly as it provides so many health benefits. This provides a great start to the day with a delicious, fibre-packed, plant oestrogen, protein and omega-3-rich plant-based breakfast. By just varying the toppings, I never get bored, even though I eat porridge most days.

Mid-morning snack – Choose from a large handful of edamame beans with lemon juice and chilli flakes/soya nuts/fresh fruit/bowl of berries/hummus with crudités/green smoothie/bowl of tofu scramble/plain soya yoghurt with fruit and nuts.

Main meal ideas – Ideally eat all your meals before 7 pm (in keeping with your circadian rhythm). Choose recipes from *Finding Me in Menopause*, our *Living PCOS Free* book and my website www.nitubajekal.com. Below are some examples of what you could enjoy in a main meal (lunch or dinner or even brunch) on a plant-predominant diet.

- Large rainbow-coloured salad, with a handful of tofu or tempeh or beans or chickpeas
- Vegetable bean/minestrone/miso soups
- Tofu/tempeh stir-fry and vegetables with wholewheat noodles
- Red lentil dal with quinoa and brown rice
- Sweet potatoes with a kidney bean stew
- Baked potatoes with baked beans and salad
- Bean burger/tempeh burger/mushroom burger and green salad
- Edamame bean spaghetti/lentil pasta with lentil ragu

Top Tip

Start all main meals with a salad (even if it is just a handful of dark green leaves and some beetroot or cherry tomatoes). Make salad a main meal, especially in the summer, and make it colourful, big and fresh. Whenever possible, try to batch cook and meal prep on a day where you have time (e.g. Sunday morning) to allow you to meet your nutrition goals.

Dr Nitu's recipes

Brunch

Salads

Mains

Curries

Rice

BRUNCH

Morning porridge oats/oatmeal

Serves 1

INGREDIENTS

3 heaped tbsp of steel-cut oats (sometimes called pinhead oats)

½ cup hot water

1 cup (200 ml) fortified unsweetened soya milk (or other plant milk if allergic to soya)

1 tsp ground cinnamon

2 tbsp flax seed powder

1 tsp milled chia seeds

Fruit (banana/apple/date/raisins and one handful of mixed fresh or frozen berries)

One handful of crushed walnuts or mixed nuts

Optional: 1 tsp unsalted peanut/almond/mixed nut butter and/or 1–2 scoops of plant protein powder

Serving suggestion: Best eaten fresh but batch cooking to save time is great too.

INSTRUCTIONS

Soak dry porridge oats in ½ cup of hot water for 15–20 minutes in a saucepan. Then add the soya milk and cook slowly until soft and creamy on stove for at least 10–12 minutes, initially bringing to a boil and then on low, stirring regularly. Add more water if needed.

Next, remove from heat and pour into a bowl. Allow it to cool for a minute or so. Now add the rest of the ingredients, mix well and enjoy.

Top Tips

Porridge oats are rich in heart-healthy soluble fibre (beta-glucans), helping to lower cholesterol levels and stabilize blood sugar levels.

Flaxseeds are a rich source of lignans (plant oestrogens) and help to reduce breast cancer risk, but are also a good source of healthy omega-3 fats, as are chia and hemp seeds. Flaxseeds need to be ground or milled for their benefits. You can mill flaxseeds and chia seeds in a coffee grinder or blender and store in an airtight jar for two weeks or so at a time. For larger batches, store in the fridge or freezer to prevent their delicate oils from going rancid.

Note: If you do not have time, you can use rolled oats instead of steel-cut oats and follow the same steps or cook in the microwave for a couple of minutes at around 900–1000 W. To add natural sweetness, mash half a banana into the oats as they cook.

You may wish to try groats, which are intact whole grain oats or buckwheat or barley for example, and have overall more fibre and nutrition. They also have a delicious nutty texture but take longer to cook. I also suggest pre-soaking overnight and batch cooking a couple of cups of groats or steel-cut oats without the milk, using just water, then store in an airtight container in the fridge and enjoy for up to four days. Add in the milk when you reheat a portion.

Sprouted grain porridge using millet or amaranth is delicious, and you can experiment with sprouting as you become more familiar with these nutritious grains.

'Feel good' protein smoothie

Serves 2

INGREDIENTS

1 medium-sized banana

1 medium-sized apple with skin

1 cup of mixed frozen berries

1 large handful of kale

1 large handful of spinach

1 tbsp each of flax and chia seeds

2 tbsp sunflower/hemp/pumpkin seeds

1 tsp cinnamon powder

4 tbsp plant protein powder (pea/hemp/brown rice) (optional)

1 peeled lime or lemon

A few sprigs of fresh or frozen mint leaves

1 small 2.5 cm piece of ginger

1 small 2.5 cm piece of turmeric root (or sub 1 tsp turmeric powder)

2 pitted dried dates

1 tbsp unsalted peanut or almond butter

½ cup uncooked rolled oats

1 litre cold water or plant milk and ice to taste

Serving suggestion: Serve cold or at room temperature.

INSTRUCTIONS

Add all the ingredients to the water and blend until smooth in a strong blender. Add more water or milk if needed and serve cold. You can also serve it thick and have it in a bowl with a spoon, dressing it with some granola or fresh chopped fruit and nuts.

Sip or chew your smoothie slowly rather than glugging it down to allow for salivary digestion in your mouth to start. Remember to rinse your mouth with water afterwards protect the enamel of your teeth.

Add silken tofu or ½ a cup of frozen peas for a protein boost instead of the protein powder.

All greens and fruits, spices and herbs can be fresh or frozen, the latter often having more nutritional value.

Smoothies are a great addition to your diet, especially if you are busy or if you are struggling to get your fruit and vegetables in.

Note: I suggest experimenting with different ingredients. Consider using a variety of seasonal fruit such as strawberries, kiwi and mangos. I tend not to overthink it and just use whatever I have around.

Golden tofu scramble

Serves 2–4

INGREDIENTS

400 g block of firm tofu

1 tsp–1 tbsp avocado or olive oil (EVVO) (optional)

1 tsp of dried basil

1 tsp cumin seeds or cumin powder

1 tsp turmeric powder

¼ tsp pepper powder

1 large finely chopped onion

1–2 finely chopped green chillies (optional)

1 chopped large red/yellow pepper

2 chopped medium-sized tomatoes

1 cup frozen or fresh green peas

1 cup fresh spinach/kale or one cube frozen spinach

1–2 tbsp soy or tamari (gluten-free) sauce

½ tsp kala namak (black salt) for eggy sulphurous taste (optional)

1 tbsp tomato paste or tomato ketchup or sriracha (optional)

Fresh basil or coriander (cilantro) leaves for garnish

INSTRUCTIONS

In a hot pan, dry roast the basil, turmeric and cumin until you can smell the spices. You can use gently heated oil to roast the spices. Avoid burning spices to reduce harmful AGEs (see 'Top tips' below).

Add the onion and chillies and sauté until pink and translucent, usually 5 minutes.

Add a tbsp or two of hot water instead of oil to cook the onion if needed. Add pepper and tomatoes, sauté for 3–4 minutes.

Add frozen peas and frozen spinach, cover and cook for 4–5 minutes on medium heat.

Grate or crumble the tofu in a separate dish. Squeeze out most of the water and add it to the pan.

Add the soy sauce, black pepper and black salt. Cook for 5 minutes, mixing thoroughly.

Add the fresh spinach now if using, and a teaspoon of ketchup/tomato paste and mix.

Garnish with herbs.

Serving suggestion: Enjoy on its own, as a side dish or in a wholemeal wrap or on sourdough or rye bread.

Top Tips

Tofu is a minimally processed product made from soya beans and is a complete protein, with vitamins, fibre and healthy plant oestrogens. Choose the organic calcium-fortified product if you can. Read more about the benefits and safety of soya in Chapter 14.

Soya can help strengthen bones and, when eaten regularly, can help reduce troublesome hot flushes in perimenopause and menopause.

The golden colour of the tofu scramble is from the curcumin, the bright golden-yellow pigment in turmeric powder that has been most studied. This phytochemical is considered to have anti-inflammatory, anti-cancer and antioxidant properties and may have a beneficial role to play in lung disease, Alzheimer's disease, arthritis and skin conditions.

The ingredient piperine in pepper helps to increase the bioavailability of turmeric. Even just a little pinch of pepper (1/20th of a tsp) can significantly boost levels.

Avoid burning spices as blackened foods and deep-frying increase toxic products called AGEs (advanced glycation end products) which cause damage to blood vessels and other tissues, including ovaries.

Dr Rajiv's tofu 'egg' sandwich filling

Serves 8 (on open-faced slices of bread)

INGREDIENTS

1 pack (400 g) firm tofu

1 pack silken tofu

1 tsp freshly ground black pepper

1 tsp smoked paprika

1 tsp garlic powder

½ tsp gochugaru (or 1 tbsp sweet paprika and 1.5 tbsp chilli powder/cayenne powder)

½ tsp English mustard

Red chilli flakes to taste

½ tsp black salt (kala namak) for the eggy flavour

Pickled onions (1 finely chopped red onion, 4 tbsp cider vinegar, 2 tbsp red wine vinegar, 1 tsp brown sugar)

INSTRUCTIONS

Choose firm tofu for this (a calcium-set tofu has the most nutrition) but avoid pressing it, as the liquid helps create the right texture.

Crumble the firm tofu in your hands, leaving a few lumps to recreate an egg salad texture.

Mix together the silken tofu with the rest of the ingredients in a large mixing bowl, stirring to combine. Mix in the crumbled tofu. Give it a taste and adjust the seasoning to your preference.

Refrigerate and enjoy leftovers within 3–4 days.

Serving suggestion: Enjoy as an open-faced sandwich on either rye bread or sourdough, topped with pickled onions, cress and crunchy vegetables such as radish or with pea shoots.

Serve with new potatoes and a salad for a light summer meal or picnic.

Top Tips

Did you know that tofu contains around 3.5 times less saturated fat than eggs, while being a fantastic source of micronutrients including protein, iron and calcium?

Try to use a tofu which is calcium-fortified (it will mention calcium in the ingredients list).

Unprocessed or minimally processed soya is a great addition to our daily diet and is beneficial for all ages and genders (unless you are in the small minority with an allergy). This is a great recipe that takes just a few minutes to prepare.

Note: Kala namak (black salt) can be found online or in Indian stores. Use regular salt if you don't have it, but you won't have the sulphuric eggy taste.

Omit the mustard and red chilli flakes for children or those sensitive to spice.

Rohini's strawberry chia pudding

Serves 2

INGREDIENTS

3 tbsp chia seeds

200 ml soya milk

1 tsp maple syrup

8 goji berries

6 strawberries

cacao nibs/walnuts (optional)

INSTRUCTIONS

Mix together chia seeds, soya milk, maple syrup and goji berries in a regular sized bowl. Let sit for a few minutes then stir again so the chia seeds don't clump together. Divide it into two equal portions in a glass or bowl.

Refrigerate for at least four hours or overnight.

Dice the strawberries and add them on top with optional cacao nibs/walnuts.

Serving suggestion: Serve cold with toppings, if desired.

Top Tips

A single tablespoon of chia seeds contains around 6 g of fibre.

Adults in the UK are recommended to get 30 g of dietary fibre each day for the general health benefits. The latest figures suggest that the average fibre intake for adults in the UK is around 17 g, far lower than what it should be.

Fibre is only found in plants

Fibre in our diet is important not just for aiding digestion and preventing constipation, but for several other health benefits. Fibre helps to maintain a healthy body weight and lowers our risks of type 2 diabetes, heart disease and certain cancers such as bowel cancer. Fibre is also important for hormonal health.

When added to water, the soluble fibre in chia seeds absorbs water (roughly 10 times their volume), which makes them swell up and form a gel in minutes. This can be satiating especially when consumed in a chia pudding with some fruit and nuts. The soluble fibre in chia seeds feeds healthy bacteria in the gut and can help regulate blood sugar and lower LDL ('bad') cholesterol. Chia seeds are small but nutritional powerhouses along with other types of seeds. They are a source of protein, calcium, iron, magnesium, zinc and niacin and a rich source of antioxidants.

Note: Optional: a teaspoon of raw cacao nibs on each pudding adds a wonderful crunch (and extra heart-healthy flavanols), or alternatively a couple of crushed walnuts.

For a richer feel, use coconut milk.

You can vary the toppings – granola, kiwi fruit, passionfruit and raspberries are some of my favourites.

SALADS

Raw yellow moong dal and cucumber salad

Serves 4

INGREDIENTS

80 g or 1 handful yellow moong dal (yellow petite lentils)

1 medium-sized cucumber chopped fine, unpeeled

½ lemon, juiced

1 tbsp fresh mint leaves or coriander (cilantro), chopped fine

1 tsp extra virgin olive oil

1 small green chilli, chopped fine

1 tsp black mustard seeds

1 tsp fresh curry leaves (optional)

INSTRUCTIONS

Rinse and soak the raw dal in a small bowl of water for one hour. Drain the water.

Heat the oil in a small pan and add the mustard seeds, chopped chilli and curry leaves.

Remove from heat when you hear the mustard seeds splutter.

Add the tempered oil mix, lemon juice, fresh mint or coriander (cilantro) and dal to the cucumber and mix thoroughly.

Serving suggestion: A refreshing salad to have as a side with a curry and rice or on its own.

Top Tips

Raw salads can add a vibrancy to main meals, as well as bringing in a variety of vitamins that may be reduced during cooking.

Use herbs, spices, flavoured vinegars and lemon juice as alternatives to salt.

Tomato and onion salad

Serves 4

INGREDIENTS

2 firm medium or large tomatoes, chopped into long slices

1 medium white onion, peeled, washed and chopped into long thin slices

1–2 handfuls sprouted mung beans (optional)

1 tbsp fresh chopped coriander (cilantro)

2 tbsp chopped jalapeños or a finely chopped green chilli

1 tbsp lemon juice and a pinch of salt

INSTRUCTIONS

Mix all ingredients together and enjoy.

Serving suggestion: Best as a side with a main meal.

Top Tips

Onions are from the allium family and have a great nutrition profile, rich in antioxidants, helping to reduce chronic inflammation, the driver of all chronic disease, such as type 2 diabetes, hypertension and heart disease.

I find washing onions (after peeling) under running water before chopping does not make my eyes water and also takes away that pungent taste in a salad.

Beetroot with rocket (arugula) salad

Serves 2

INGREDIENTS

80–100 g or 1 bag rocket (arugula) or colourful mixed salad leaves

3 cooked beetroots, chopped into thin slices or 1 cm cubes

a handful of crushed walnuts and sunflower seeds

a large glug of balsamic vinegar

Serving suggestion: Serve cold.

INSTRUCTIONS

Mix it all together and serve as a side or starter salad.

Sweetcorn or cucumber mint raita

Serves 4

INGREDIENTS

1 small can or 250 g cooked sweet corn

or ½ large or 1 medium cucumber grated

250 ml soya yoghurt (or other plant milk yoghurt)

50 ml soya or plant milk

1 tbsp garden mint sauce or 1 tbsp finely chopped fresh mint or
1 tsp fresh cumin and pepper powder

INSTRUCTIONS

Whip the soya yoghurt to a smooth consistency with the soya milk and mint sauce.

Add the sweetcorn or grated cucumber and a pinch of salt if you wish.

Serving suggestion: Serve cold as a side. Tastes wonderful with tofu vegetable rice.

Top Tips

Sweetcorn is a complex starchy carbohydrate that allows regulation of our blood sugars slowly and is full of fibre.

Soya yoghurt is nutritious and tasty, and can be made easily at home from soya milk, with a plant-based yoghurt starter kit bought online.

Adding herbs and spices (mint, pepper and cumin) to any dish adds flavour and increases the antioxidant power of a dish significantly.

Beetroot pomegranate pearl hummus

Serves 2–4

INGREDIENTS

2 cans (800 g) or 3 cups cooked chickpeas

100 ml chickpea water (aquafaba)

3 medium garlic cloves

2 tbsp tahini (sesame seed paste)

2 cooked beetroots chopped

4 tbsp fresh pomegranate pearls

½ tsp paprika

1 handful walnuts

½ tsp black pepper

salt to taste

juice of 3 medium lemons

1–2 tbsp extra virgin olive oil (optional)

INSTRUCTIONS

Soak the dried chickpeas overnight. Rinse thoroughly.

You may wish to sprout the chickpeas. Sprout in a sprout maker or in a warm place for 24–48 hours, until you see the white tails. Sprouting increases bioavailability of vitamins and makes chickpeas even more of a powerhouse. Rinse thoroughly again before cooking.

Cook the chickpeas until really soft (use a pressure cooker or an instant pot), or simply use 2 cans of chickpeas (800 g).

Use a strong blender and add the ingredients one at a time to the chickpeas and chickpea water and use a pulsing action initially and then blend at low.

The aquafaba water is the chickpea water from just one can, or from the cooked chickpea water. Add more aquafaba if you want the hummus to be a thinner consistency.

Blend high speed for a few seconds only at the end, adding the lemon juice and optional olive oil at this stage.

Garnish with the remaining pomegranate pearls and the paprika.

Serving suggestion: Enjoy on salads and in wraps or as a dip.

Top Tips

All long-living societies include legumes every day in their diet. Legumes include chickpeas, beans, lentils, soybeans, black-eyed peas and sugar snap/snow/green peas.

Aquafaba is the viscous water in which chickpeas have been cooked. You can use it as egg replacer in desserts too.

Easy kimchi by The Happy Pear

For those who do not know what kimchi is, it is a Korean-style sauerkraut with a wonderful spicy tangy gingery flavour. It is packed full of probiotics great for digestion and the immune system. This recipe was developed by Fiona, our wonderful fermenter, through lots of experimenting. Traditionally kimchi is made using Chinese cabbage, but we adapted to make it quicker and easier and still taste fab! It is great to make in a big batch as it lasts for a long time, and the longer you let it ferment, the flavours just get more developed. This does take time to make, but it's so worth it.

Serves 1

INGREDIENTS

1 kg mixed veg such as carrot, pak choi, Chinese cabbage, radish, leek, beet

20 g salt

Sauce

4 tbsp tamari

1 tsp maple syrup

25 g rice flour

200 ml water

5 cloves garlic

½ onion

½ tsp kelp powder

2½ tbsp gochugaru (or 1 tbsp sweet paprika and 1½ tbsp chilli powder/cayenne powder)

INSTRUCTIONS

Roughly chop the vegetables into bite-sized pieces. Put in a large bowl or saucepan and add the salt. Mix well and bash with a potato masher or saucer for 2 minutes. Leave to sit for 1–2 hours or even overnight.

Rinse and wash the salt away and put back in the bowl/saucepan.

Peel the garlic cloves. Add the ingredients for the sauce and blend till smooth. Pour over the already salted veg. Now add the gochugaru or paprika/chilli mix and mix well.

Add this mix into a large sterile mason jar with a lid for fermentation. Ensure the vegetables are submerged under the sauce and natural vegetable juices, as this is a lactic acid fermentation process. Leave to ferment on the counter for 2–3 days, until it starts to become bubbly. Taste and if you prefer it to be more acidic, leave for longer. The longer you leave it to ferment at room temperature, the more acidic it will become. Once you are happy with the level of acidity, put the jar in the fridge and enjoy for many months or years to follow.

Top Tips

Adding fermented foods, such as sauerkraut, kimchi and pickled vegetables, to your daily diet can help your gut microbiome flourish.

This is a 2 per cent salt solution method which makes it super easy to adapt to whatever volume of veg or even fruit you are fermenting. This basic method is applied when fermenting any fruit or veg. You can add some flavour agents such as garlic, ginger, turmeric, cumin, chilli and herbs or spices to give each ferment more personality. We kept this one simple, just so you know how it's done.

Note: Check on your kimchi every few days, to make sure that the vegetables stays submerged in the liquid. Sometimes, the top layer that is exposed to the air can start to go off slightly but don't worry about this, it can simply be scraped off and the underneath layer should still be perfectly fine to eat. Time and temperature are the two secret ingredients for fermentation: the longer you leave it to ferment, the stronger and more acidic the flavour, and the warmer the temperature, the quicker it will ferment.

MAINS

Quinestrone soup

Serves 6

INGREDIENTS

3 litres water (or 3 litres homemade vegetable stock, if not using stock cubes)

2 small low salt vegan stock cubes (optional)

1 tbsp dried basil

1 large onion finely chopped

garlic cloves crushed and chopped fine

2 green chillies slit lengthways

1 can (400 g) chopped tomatoes (double the amount if using fresh tomatoes)

4 fresh large tomatoes, diced

2 potatoes, diced into small cubes (1 cm)

2 carrots, diced into small cubes (1 cm)

1 large handful green beans, chopped fine

1 head broccoli into florets, diced including stalks

1 cup frozen or fresh peas

400 g can butter beans or cannellini or haricot beans (rinsed)

1 courgette (zucchini), diced into cubes (1 cm)

1½ cup quinoa rinsed

1 tsp black pepper

salt (optional)

red chilli flakes (optional)

handful of fresh basil leaves, chopped, keep aside stalks

INSTRUCTIONS

In a large pan, add 3 litres of boiling water. Add the stock cubes, dried basil, chopped onion, garlic, chillies, both canned and fresh tomatoes and chopped basil stalks for flavour, and bring to boil.

Keep chopping vegetables and adding as you go along. Add potatoes and carrots first, as they take longer to cook. Keep the pan covered and on medium heat.

After approximately 10 minutes, add the beans, broccoli, peas, can of butter beans, courgette and quinoa. Add some more hot water if you feel the need.

Bring to the boil and then cover and simmer for 30 minutes. Check the potatoes are cooked.

Season to taste with salt and pepper. Add basil as a garnish and sprinkle on red chilli flakes if you like the heat.

Serving suggestion: Serve hot with seeded rye bread or gluten-free bread or on its own. Leftovers make great next day lunches.

Top Tip

Quinoa is an ancient pseudo grain and is technically a seed. Quinoa is gluten free and is high in protein and rich in zinc, fibre and folate. Peas are legumes, to which beans and lentils also belong.

Daisy's easy beans: Louvi with courgettes and chard

Serves 4

INGREDIENTS

400 g dried black eyed beans or 3 × 400 g cans black eyed beans

1 large bunch chard or any leafy greens, chopped rough

2 large courgettes or zucchini cut into 1 cm thick rounds

1 large white onion chopped fine

4 cloves garlic chopped fine

2 tbsp extra virgin olive oil

1 tsp pepper

salt to taste

2 lemons, juiced

2 tbsp pickled jalapeños

2 tbsp chopped fresh parsley

2 tbsp chopped dill

INSTRUCTIONS

If using dried beans, ideally soak them in cold water overnight.

Boil the beans in a litre of water until soft. There will be some foam on the surface, remove with a slotted spoon. The water will look dark but when beans are nearly cooked, add the juice of a lemon and the water will turn clear.

Add the squeezed lemon into the pot for extra flavour and remove before serving.

Add the chard and courgettes. Simmer until all is cooked and soft. Season with salt and pepper.

If using canned beans, add the rinsed beans, lemon juice, chard and courgettes, salt and pepper to a litre of water and cook all until soft.

In a separate pan, sauté the chopped onion and garlic in one tbsp of the olive oil until translucent. Stir this into the cooked beans.

Make a dressing of the rest of the olive oil, chopped parsley, chopped jalapeños and the remaining lemon juice and pour over when serving.

Serving suggestion: This Greek-inspired black eyed beans, with leafy greens and courgettes, is delicious served with the dressing, and topped with a finely chopped cucumber, tomato, black olives and onion salad for crunch. Louvi can be enjoyed with some sesame seeded Greek bread.

Top Tips

This simple dish is bursting with antioxidants with the herbs, protein and fibre from the beans and is a great main dish or side.

Experiment with different types of beans as each type of bean (part of the legume family) has a different flavour and texture when cooked.

Beans are a cornerstone of the Blue Zone diet, which is a mostly plant-based diet, consisting of almost 95 per cent vegetables, fruits, grains and legumes. Ikaria in Greece is a Blue Zone, where people live to be centenarians, usually without chronic disease such as type 2 diabetes and heart disease.

The Happy Pear's pan-fried tofu with steamed greens and quinoa

Serves 2

INGREDIENTS

1½ cups or 250 g cooked quinoa

1 head pak choi (bok choy) or 100 g spinach leaves

200 g firm tofu

15 g or 1 small thumb-sized piece fresh ginger

100 g cherry tomatoes

120 g kidney beans

2 tbsp tamari

1 lime juiced

Chop the tofu block in half width-wise and then diagonally into triangle shapes.

Finely chop the ginger. Cut off the bottom of the pak choi, separate it out and give it a good wash.

Put a medium-sized non-stick pan on high heat. Once the pan is really hot, turn it down to medium and add the tofu and the ginger. Cook for 2 minutes.

Turn the tofu and cook for a further 2 minutes. If it starts to stick, add a couple of tablespoons of water. Using a wooden spoon, scrape off any of the browning and incorporate it.

Add the pak choi leaves along with 3–4 tablespoons of water and cover with a lid. Leave to steam for 2–3 minutes.

Remove the pak choi and put on the plates ready to serve.

The tofu should have started to golden on each side, add in the tamari – the pan should make a loud frying noise. Move the tofu around so that all the tofu gets a good covering from the tamari and then turn off the heat. This will take less than 1 minute.

Add the quinoa into a mixing bowl. Quarter the cherry tomatoes and add along with a pinch of salt, black pepper, the juice of the lime. Finely slice one of the pak choi leaves and add in also. Mix it all well.

Serve both plates with the tofu steaks, some steamed pak choi greens and some of the quinoa salad.

Serving suggestion: Sprinkle some nutritional yeast on top for a cheesy flavour.

Top Tips

All plants contain the nine essential amino acids that our body cannot make. There is no need to worry as long as one is eating a variety of plant foods.

The added advantage of plant protein is that it does not come with the issues that animal protein has, such as high levels of saturated fat, organic pollutants and a bigger carbon footprint (whether organic, grass fed or factory farmed).

This complete dish has two high-quality plant protein sources in tofu and quinoa.

Pepper mushroom wrap

INGREDIENTS

500 g chestnut or button mushrooms chopped into halves

1 tbsp extra virgin olive oil or canola oil (optional)

1 tsp cumin powder

1 tsp pepper powder

¼ tsp of asafoetida (hing) (optional)

2 slit fresh green chillies or chopped fine

small cup frozen or fresh peas

salt to taste

fresh basil or coriander or parsley leaves for garnish

INSTRUCTIONS

In a heated pan, add the spices and the green chillies to gently heated oil, taking care not to burn the spices.

Add in the mushrooms and sauté for a couple of minutes on high heat, mixing in the spices.

Cover and let it cook on low heat for 10 minutes. Mushrooms tend to release water so allow to cook in their own water.

Add the frozen or fresh peas, mix thoroughly, cover and cook for 5 minutes. Remove the lid and cook for another 5 minutes on medium heat to allow the water to evaporate.

Garnish with herbs after turning off the heat. Add a squeeze of lemon to cut back on salt.

Serving suggestion: Serve in a wrap with crunchy peppers and green leaves or serve warm as a side with a main meal or on top of a salad.

Top Tips

Mushrooms are best and safest eaten cooked.

Using olive oil in this dish helps to increase antioxidant activity of mushrooms.

You can increase the vitamin D content of mushrooms by exposing them to direct sunlight for about an hour. When fresh button mushrooms are deliberately exposed to midday sunlight for 15–120 minutes, depending on the strength of the sun, they generate significant amounts of vitamin D2, usually in excess of 10 µg/100 g. However, do remember to supplement with vitamin D, especially in the winter months, as no food is reliable enough for us to meet all our daily vitamin D requirement.

Mushrooms also contain beta-glucans, which boost immune response. Eating even a single small button mushroom a day (less than 10 g) has been shown to help reduce the risk of breast cancer.

Mushrooms contain dietary fibre, protein, amino acids, vitamins and trace minerals, and are naturally low in fat and calories.

CURRIES

The Happy Pear's Vietnamese sweet potato and tempeh curry
Serves 2

INGREDIENTS

750 g sweet potato

200 g tempeh (if not available substitute with firm tofu/mushrooms)

400 ml tin low-fat coconut milk (ensure low fat)

200 ml vegetable stock

1 small 2.5 cm piece of fresh ginger

2 cloves garlic

juice of 1 lime

1 tbsp maple syrup

1 tbsp curry powder

1 tsp salt

2 tbsp tamari/soy sauce

3 scallions/spring onions

½ a head pak choi

small bunch fresh coriander (cilantro) leaves, chopped

INSTRUCTIONS

Preheat the oven to 180°C/350°F/gas mark 4.

Peel and finely chop the garlic and ginger. Finely slice the scallions.

Chop the sweet potatoes into bite-sized pieces (leaving the skin as this is where a lot of the fibre and nutrients are).

Place the sweet potato on a baking tray with a decent pinch of salt and bake in the preheated oven for 20 minutes.

Mix the tin of low-fat coconut milk together with chopped ginger, chopped garlic, lime juice, maple syrup, curry powder, tamari/soy sauce and the 200 ml vegetable stock into a blender and whiz until everything is smooth.

Dice up the tempeh into small-sized cubes (around 1½ cm) – the smaller they are, the more flavour each piece will have. Put the diced tempeh onto a baking tray and dress with approximately half of the dressing. Mixing the tempeh and the sauce well is important to make sure each piece is full of flavour.

Put the tempeh into the preheated oven and bake for 15 minutes. After 10 minutes, stir the tempeh to ensure that the dressing is well spread.

Meanwhile, pour in the other half of the dressing in a large-sized saucepan – this will become the sauce of the dish along with any remaining sauce from the baked tempeh dish. Put on a high heat and bring to the boil, then reduce to a simmer.

Once the tempeh and sweet potato are done, transfer them into the pot with the simmering sauce and mix well.

Simply bring the dish to a boil and then reduce to a simmer. Chop off the end of the pak choi and finely chop the full length of it. Do the same with the scallions and add both to the dish. Cook for a further 2 minutes, then remove from the heat.

Serving suggestion: This curry goes great with wholewheat noodles, brown rice or wholemeal couscous.

Top Tip

Tempeh is a fermented food, made of mainly soya beans, and is a nutritious, affordable and sustainable high-quality source of protein. Rich in isoflavones or plant oestrogens, it is a helpful addition to one's diet to help perimenopause and menopause. Regular intake of tempeh is good for the heart. For more information on soya, please see Chapter 14.

Note: If you can't source tempeh, use tofu instead, and if you cannot find either, simply use some sort of mushrooms instead.

Replace the garlic with the green part of three scallions and use just the green part of the scallions in the recipe, if bloating from garlic is an issue for you.

Red kidney bean sweet potato curry

Serves 6

INGREDIENTS

3 × 400g cans red kidney beans, rinsed (or 400 g cooked from dried beans)

3 medium-sized red onions, peeled and chopped fine

5 cm large piece fresh ginger root, grated fine

6 large cloves garlic, grated

4 green chillies, chopped fine or slit long

4 large fresh tomatoes, chopped fine

400 g can chopped tomatoes or double the fresh tomatoes

2 large, sweet potatoes, chopped into 1½ cm cubes (unpeeled, washed)

200 g or large bag fresh chopped kale or spinach, frozen is fine

1 small bunch fresh coriander (cilantro) leaves (stalks finely chopped)

1 tsp EACH cumin seeds, ground cumin, ground coriander, chilli powder, turmeric powder

¼ tsp asafoetida (hing) (optional)

¼ tsp ground pepper powder

¼ tsp brown sugar or jaggery

1 tbsp amchoor (dried mango) powder or pomegranate powder (anardana powder) – optional

2–3 cups of hot water

1 tbsp extra virgin olive or rapeseed oil (optional)

1 lemon, juiced

salt to taste

INSTRUCTIONS

In a heated large pan, dry roast all the spices or in gently heated oil, except the amchoor or pomegranate powder, until you get the aroma, taking care not to burn the spices.

Add the chopped onions, chillies, ginger and garlic, and sauté for 3–4 minutes on a high heat mixing thoroughly.

Add a few splashes of hot water and sauté for 5 minutes.

Add the chopped and canned tomatoes, sugar, coriander stalks and the amchoor or anardana powder. Mix thoroughly and cook for another 5 minutes.

Add the sweet potato cubes, cover and cook on low heat for about 15 minutes.

Add the rinsed beans, a couple of cups of hot water, mix thoroughly and cover and cook for another 15 minutes. Add frozen spinach now if using. Check sweet potatoes are cooked through.

Add the fresh kale or spinach, cover and switch heat off and let spinach cook in the heat.

Mix in the lemon juice and garnish with coriander leaves.

Serving suggestion: Serve with brown or red rice with cucumber or sweetcorn raita and a side salad or on its own like a stew or with bread/flatbread.

Top Tips

Be bold with spices for maximum flavour and health benefits.

Beans contain plant oestrogens (phytoestrogens) that help reduce menopausal hot flushes when eaten regularly.

Complex starchy carbohydrates such as sweet potatoes or potatoes in their skin and beans are full of gut health promoting fibre and vitamins.

Choose red onions over white onions as they have more antioxidants and flavonoids, which have anti-inflammatory and anti-cancer properties.

Crushing or chopping garlic releases alliinase, an enzyme that helps in the formation of allicin, a healthy organic sulphur compound that reduces inflammation and has anti-cancer properties. After crushing, leave the garlic for ten minutes before cooking or storing in the freezer, to allow for maximum benefit.

Rustic buttery black dal
(Dhaba style)
Serves 6

This black dal (split gram lentil or chilke wali urad dal) is bursting with flavour, has a creamy luxurious taste, very different in texture and taste to the more commonly cooked lentils. This is my take on this ancient and famous dish from the north of India. It is often served with hot chappatis in roadside food stalls called dhabas. This dish takes time to cook but it is so worth it.

INGREDIENTS

Split black gram lentils: 2 cups dry weight or 500g, wash and rinse a few times and soak in water for a few hours

2 red onions, chopped fine

3–4 green chillies chopped fine

5 cm large piece of fresh ginger, grated fine

4 garlic cloves, grated

4 medium fresh tomatoes

400 g can tomatoes (or double fresh tomatoes)

200 g spinach or kale (fresh or frozen)

1 tbsp extra virgin olive oil (optional)

1 tsp turmeric

¼ tsp asafoetida (hing) (optional)

1 tbsp coriander powder

1 tbsp cumin powder

1 tbsp cumin seeds

1 tsp red chilli powder (optional)

1 tbsp pomegranate (anardana) powder (optional)

salt to taste

½ tsp brown sugar or jaggery

1 lemon, juiced

fresh coriander (cilantro) leaves and stalks finely chopped: large handful

1 tbsp vegan butter and/or 50 ml vegan cream (optional)

Serving suggestion: Serve with flatbread or rice and a mint raita or as a soup with a large dollop of soya Greek yoghurt or other plant yoghurt.

INSTRUCTIONS

In a heated deep pan, dry roast the spices (cumin, coriander) or roast in oil, taking care to avoid burning the spices to reduce harmful AGEs.

Add the chopped onion, garlic, ginger and chillies and sauté on high heat for 2–3 minutes, allowing the onions to sweat. Keep stirring, so it doesn't catch at the bottom.

Add 4–5 tbsp of hot water and cook the onions until soft for another 5 minutes on medium heat. Keep stirring.

Add the chilli powder, turmeric, pomegranate powder, asafoetida and brown sugar and mix.

Now add all the chopped tomatoes and coriander stalks and cook on low heat for 10 minutes.

Add the washed lentils and about 6–8 cups of hot water (2–3 times). Bring to boil and cook on a low flame until soft for at least 45 minutes. Add frozen spinach now if using.

To get that really creamy texture, cook on low heat for another 30–60 minutes.

Add the fresh spinach or kale in just a minute before turning the heat off.
Add the vegan butter now and stir it in.
Garnish with lemon juice and coriander.
Swirl the vegan cream on the top.

Top Tips

You can use an instant pot too for this recipe to save time.

Legumes form part of all long-living societies, providing starchy complex carbohydrates so important for glycaemic control, rich in fibre, micronutrients and vitamins.

Try to eat 2–3 portions of legumes a day. A portion is only a handful or 80 g and is easily achieved.

Ginger is a 'root', or the rhizome, of the plant *Zingiber officinale*. It is native to Asia where it has been used as a spice for over 4400 years. Ginger is related to turmeric, which also has powerful health benefits. Ginger has been prized for its medicinal purposes (mostly due to gingerol, a natural component of ginger root) for thousands of years.

Ginger may have a role in immune support and reducing inflammation in the gut. As a result of its benefits in reducing inflammation, it may also benefit osteoarthritis and joint pain.

Note: Be bold with spices and slow cook this dal to allow flavours to come through.

Tea-infused spicy chickpeas

Serves 4

INGREDIENTS

2 × 400g cans chickpeas (washed and rinsed), or cook from dried (rinse and soak overnight and cook until very soft)

1–2 fresh green chillies, slit

5 cm large piece fresh ginger, grated fine

1 tsp fresh cumin powder

1 tsp cumin seeds

¼ tsp asafoetida (hing), optional

2 black teabags (English Breakfast or other)

250 ml boiling water

fresh coriander (cilantro) leaves to garnish

1 lemon, juiced

salt to taste

1 tsp olive oil

INSTRUCTIONS

In a pan, heat the olive oil and add the cumin seeds, cumin powder and asafoetida powder (hing) to help with bloating, taking care to avoid burning the spices.

Almost immediately, add the cooked chickpeas and the boiling water to just cover the chickpeas.

Toss in the green chillies, grated ginger and bring to the boil.

Simmer for about 10 minutes. With the back of the spoon, crush some of the peas into the water to thicken it slightly and give it a rustic look.

Add in the teabags (gives it a lovely flavour and dark colour) and cook for another 10–15 minutes on low heat. Remove before serving.

Add the coriander leaves and lemon juice and add salt to taste.

Serving suggestion: Eat as a side or on its own. Can be eaten hot or cold.

Top Tips

You can use an instant pot or pressure cooker to make this dish.

Legumes (beans, peas, lentils, pulses) are the staple of all long living societies.

If you feel bloated with legumes, this will soon settle. You will notice as you cut animal products from your diet, healthy gut bacteria that deal with fibre and digestion of beans and vegetables start flourishing. Introduce beans in small amounts and make sure they are cooked until really soft (you should be able to mash the peas with the back of a fork).

Chickpeas are versatile and can be used in sweet and savoury dishes. A variety of lentils is available very cheap in most ethnic shops. Freezing chickpeas dishes works well.

Hummus, chickpea flour and aquafaba can be used in a variety of dishes.

Chickpeas can be sprouted too and added to salads, increasing the vitamin and antioxidant content. Chickpeas are a great source of soluble fibre and phytoestrogens as well as a good source of vitamins, especially folate, B vitamins, iron and phosphorus.

Cumin has many benefits for health as do most herbs and spices. Cumin seeds and powder can help with digestion, weight loss, blood sugar and cholesterol control.

Cabbage jhunka

Konkani South Indian style sabji with gram flour (split brown chickpea flour)

Serves 4

INGREDIENTS

1 small to medium white cabbage, chopped fine

2 medium red or white onions, chopped fine

3 green chillies, slit long or chopped fine

1 tbsp olive oil (optional)

1 tsp turmeric powder

2 tsp mustard seeds

¼ tsp asafoetida (hing) (optional)

1 tbsp fresh or dried curry leaves

4 heaped tbsp gram flour (besan)

salt to taste

1 large bunch of chopped fresh coriander (cilantro) (use stems too)

INSTRUCTIONS

Wash the cabbage and remove just the very outer leaves, but only if needed.

Chop the cabbage, onions and chillies finely and keep separate.

Roast the spices in a heated pan until you hear the mustard seeds spluttering (use gently heated olive oil if you prefer).

Add the onions and green chillies, and cook down until pink, adding 4–5 tbsp of hot water to cook the onions. Now add the gram flour and roast constantly for 2–3 minutes on a medium heat, taking care not to burn the flour.

Now add another couple of tbsp of hot water. Add the chopped cabbage with the coriander stems. Mix in thoroughly until the besan (gram flour) coats the cabbage.

Cook on a high heat for a couple of minutes, then cover with a lid. Cook on low flame for 10–15 minutes, checking halfway to see if cabbage has softened. You do not want it too crunchy or too mushy, as you want the flavours to burst through.

Serving suggestion: Eat as a side dish with dal and rice, in a wrap with salad leaves or with rotis/naan.

Top Tips

Cabbage belongs to the cruciferous brassica family, same as broccoli, cauliflower, kale, collard greens and brussels sprouts. This entire family is great for heart health. If bloating is an issue for you with the brassica family, this dish may not be for you.

Cabbage contains phytochemicals including isothiocyanates and glucosinolates. Boiling reduces the levels of cauliflower glucosinolates, while other cooking methods, such as steaming, microwaving and stir frying, have no significant effect on the levels.

The besan or gram flour gives this dish an extra protein boost, making this dish delicious. Gram flour is made from split brown chickpeas while chickpea flour is made from regular chickpeas (garbanzo beans).

Coriander is a key ingredient in this dish. Try adding herbs and spices to every meal because of their powerful antioxidant anti-inflammatory properties.

Avoid burning spices as blackened foods and deep-frying increase toxic products called AGEs (advanced glycation end products) which cause damage to blood vessels and other tissues, including ovaries.

Animal foods, especially barbecued meat, have the highest level of AGEs. Grilled and even poached chicken has significantly more AGEs than fried potatoes. Steaming and boiling create the least AGEs in food.

RICE

Cooking brown rice

Serves 4–6

INGREDIENTS

3 cups brown rice

6 cups water

INSTRUCTIONS

Thoroughly rinse the brown rice in a sieve.

Add to the stove, bring to the boil and then lower to simmer.

Cook for around 20 minutes with the lid on, on a low heat, checking occasionally.

Eat immediately or cool quickly and then refrigerate (eat within a couple of days).

Top Tips

Rice can be a satiating and healthy addition to the diet and is a good source of energy, has little fat and has some protein too.

Ideally, choose brown or red rice, as there are more nutrients and fibre than in white rice.

Cook with equal parts of quinoa to add a further protein and fibre boost.

Cooking red rice and quinoa

Serves 4–6

INGREDIENTS

1 cup red rice

1 cup quinoa

5–6 cups water

INSTRUCTIONS

Thoroughly rinse the red rice and quinoa in a sieve.

Add to the stove, bring to the boil and then lower to simmer.

Cook for around 30–40 minutes with the lid on, on a low heat, checking occasionally if more water is needed. Check rice is soft as red rice takes longer to cook.

Eat immediately. If you have leftovers, cool and refrigerate (eat within a couple of days).

Top Tips

Brown and red rice have more fibre than white rice and will keep you fuller for longer.

Soaking the red rice for a few hours (then rinsing and draining) significantly reduces cooking time.

Quinoa is a pseudo grain and is a good source of high quality plant protein and fibre and contains iron and magnesium.

Tofu vegetable rice

Serves 4

INGREDIENTS

3 cups cooked brown or red rice

400 g block firm tofu cut into small 1 cm cubes

3–4 tbsp light soy sauce or tamari which is gluten-free

2 tbsp dried basil

1 tbsp extra virgin olive oil (optional)

1 large red onion, chopped finely

3–4 medium sized cloves garlic, smashed, peeled and minced finely

3–4 green chillies, deseeded, chopped as fine as you can

2 cups or 250 g mixed frozen or fresh veg (beans, peas, carrots, sweetcorn etc.)

2 tbsp tomato ketchup or sriracha sauce or tomato paste

salt to taste if needed

fresh basil leaves chopped for garnish

INSTRUCTIONS

Thoroughly rinse the 1½ cups of raw brown rice in a sieve.

Add to the stove, bring to the boil and then lower to simmer.

Cook for around 20 minutes with the lid on, on a low heat, checking occasionally.

Allow to cool and avoid rice getting too soggy.

Place a large skillet or heavy bottomed pan on a medium to high heat. When it is hot, add the tofu and dry sauté. Leave it to brown on one side before turning and this will prevent the tofu from sticking.

Halfway through, add 1 tbsp of soy sauce. Remove tofu from the heat once crispy.

In the same heated pan, add in dried basil, onion, garlic, chillies (add in optional olive oil). Add 3–4 tbsp of hot water and let it cook, stirring frequently.

Once the onions are slightly caramelized, add the frozen/fresh vegetables, mix thoroughly, increasing the heat for 3–5 minutes, then cover and cook for about 7 minutes on low heat.

Add in the rice and tofu, tomato/sriracha sauce, remaining soy sauce and mix thoroughly.

Switch off the heat, garnish with some fresh basil.

Serving suggestion: Leave to rest a few minutes before serving with a cold cucumber mint raita and a side salad (choose from above).

Top Tips

Aim to eat 80 g (a small handful) of tofu a few times a week as one of your two to four portions of soya a day. This will give you healthy protein, fibre, vitamins and healthy plant phytoestrogens.

Any rice will work – black or red rice are even more fibre rich but require longer cooking times usually.

You can put the cubed tofu on a silicone mat and bake at 400 F/180 degrees fan oven/gas mark 6 for about 20 minutes until crispy on both sides.

Cooking techniques impact the nutritional value of herbs, so if you are cooking fresh herbs such as basil for longer than around 10 minutes, some nutrients such as heat-labile vitamin C will be significantly decreased. In these situations, dried herbs come in handy.

69 per cent of UK adults are estimated to be eating too much salt, according to a National Diet and Nutrition Survey study (2020).[2] Herbs and spices flavour food without the negative health impact of too much sodium. Aside from their nutritional properties, they also make meals more delicious, flavourful and enjoyable.

Resources

Websites

Dr Nitu Bajekal MD ObGyn www.nitubajekal.com

Dr Rajiv Bajekal www.rajivbajekal.com

Rohini Bajekal Nutritionist www.rohinibajekal.com

Royal College of Obstetricians and Gynaecologists (RCOG, UK) www.rcog.org.uk

The British Menopause Society www.thebms.org.uk

The Menopause Society (North American Menopause Society (NAMS)) www.menopause.org

Australasian Menopause Society www.menopause.org.au

NICE, The National Institute for Health and Care Excellence, England Guidance (providing advice and information services for health, public health and social care professionals) www.nice.org.uk/guidance/ng23

UpToDate evidence-based clinical resource for medical and patient information www.uptodate.com/contents/menopause-beyond-the-basics

NHS (National Health Service) www.nhs.uk/conditions/menopause

Plant-Based Health Professionals (organization educating health professionals, members of the public and policy makers) https://plantbasedhealthprofessionals.com

ACLM The American College of Lifestyle Medicine https://www.lifestylemedicine.org/Scientific-Evidence

CDC (Centers for Disease Control and Prevention) https://www.cdc.gov/diabetes/basics/pcos.html

Mayo Clinic, USA www.mayoclinic.org

BDA (The Association of UK Dietitians) www.bda.uk.com

US Department of Health and Human Services https://health.gov/moveyourway

WHO (World Health Organization) https://www.who.int/news-room/fact-sheets/detail/physical-activity

Harvard School of Public Health https://www.hsph.harvard.edu/nutritionsource/healthy-eating-plate/

Menopause: Causes, Symptoms, and Treatment | Patient https://patient.info

Women's Health Initiative whi.org

Support groups

Daisy Network: a charity for women with POI (premature ovarian insufficiency) https://www.daisynetwork.org/

The Menopause Charity www.themenopausecharity.org

Black Women in Menopause: a private Facebook and events group @blackwomeninmenopause

Black Menopause And Beyond Instagram @blkmeno

Feelgoodwithlavina.com by Lavina Mehta MBE. The British South Asian PT shares accessible strength workouts, health tips and her own perimenopause experience

Download this symptom questionnaire form from the Menopause Charity: www.themenopausecharity.org/wp-content/uploads/2021/05/Symptom-Checker.pdf

Red Hot Mamas (inspire.com)

Queer/LGBTQIA+ Menopause www.queermenopause.com

Black Menopause and Beyond Podcast with Anita Powell

Early Menopause and POI advocate Sheree Hargreaves @lifeofpoi_

Books

The Menopause Guidebook, 9th edition NAMES (The North American Menopause Society) (The North American Menopause Society, 2020)

The Complete Guide to POI and Early Menopause, Dr Hannah Short and Dr Mandy Leonhardt (Sheldon Press, 2022)

Living PCOS Free, Dr Nitu Bajekal, MD FRCOG ObGyn and Rohini Bajekal (Hammersmith Health Books, 2022)

Black and Menopausal, Yansie Rolston and Yvonne Christie (Editors) (Jessica Kingsley Publishers, 2023)

Menopausing, Davina McCall with Dr Naomi Potter (HQ, 2022)

Your Body in Balance, Neal Barnard, MD (Sheldon Press, 2020)

Other

The Happy Menopause Course with The Happy Pear and Dr Nitu Bajekal (thehappypear.ie)

Glossary

A

Acupuncture: the use of ancient Chinese medicine that involves the insertion of fine needles at specific anatomical sites in the body for therapeutic or preventative purposes. This treatment is used widely in pain clinics in the UK.

Adenomyosis: where the lining of the womb pushes into the muscle layer of the womb (also known as uterine or internal endometriosis), often causing heavy and/or painful periods.

AFAB: assigned female at birth.

AGEs: advanced glycation end products. These harmful compounds are formed when protein or fat combine with sugar in the bloodstream. This process is called glycation.

Alzheimer's disease: a type of brain disorder that causes problems with memory, thinking and behaviour. This is a gradually progressive condition and the most common form of dementia in the UK.

Amenorrhea: absence of periods during the reproductive years of life. Medical advice should be sought if more than three months of missing a period or earlier if concerned.

AMH or anti-Mullerian hormone: a marker of ovarian egg reserve, often used in fertility workups, falling to very low levels a few years before the onset of menopause.

Androgens: hormones involved in the development and maintenance of male secondary sexual characteristics and structures. In women, they have an important role to play in the production of oestrogen and in maintaining muscle and bone mass, sexual function and wellbeing. Testosterone, dehydroepiandrosterone (DHEA), androstenedione are some of the important androgens produced by the ovaries and adrenal glands in women.

Anovulation: failure to release an egg from the ovary.

Antioxidant: substance that inhibits oxidation (for example, vitamin C or E) and removes potentially damaging oxidizing agents in a living organism.

Assigned female at birth (AFAB): when a person's gender identity is different from the female sex they were assigned at birth.

Atrophic vaginitis: or vaginal atrophy is a condition, most commonly seen in menopause, arising from a lack of oestrogen causing the vaginal skin to become thinner, pale, dry and inflamed.

B

Benign: non-cancerous.

Bioidentical HRT: artificial hormones, usually made from plants that are chemically similar to those produced by the human body. Compounded bioidentical hormone replacement therapy or cBHRT does not follow the strict regulation and licensing required by conventional HRT. Due to lack of evidence for their safety and efficacy, these custom compounded 'bioidentical hormones' are not recommended by medical experts worldwide.

Biopsy: a tissue specimen removed and examined microscopically for the presence of disease (often cancer), for example endometrial biopsy.

Blood pressure (BP): recorded as two numbers. The first (top) number is 'systolic blood pressure', which measures how much pressure your blood exerts on the artery walls when the heart beats. The second (bottom) number is 'diastolic blood pressure', which is the amount of pressure exerted on your artery walls while your heart is resting between beats. Optimal blood pressure is less than 120/80 mm Hg.

Blue Zones: geographic areas where people have low rates of chronic disease and live longer than anywhere else. Examples are Sardinia, Italy, Okinawa, Japan and Loma Linda in California, USA.

Body identical HRT: man-made hormones, extracted from plants and chemically similar to those produced by the human body. Regulated bioidentical hormone replacement therapy (rBHRT) is often referred to as body identical HRT. The difference from compounded bioidentical HRT is that body identical HRT is regulated and approved by medical experts.

Body mass index (BMI): measure based on a person's weight and height to estimate if a person is at a healthy weight, overweight, or obese. A BMI of 18–24.9 is considered a healthy weight, 25–29.9 is considered overweight, and 30 or higher is considered obese. It is an imperfect measure, but since women in perimenopause and menopause may be at risk for excess weight and its complications, health providers look to the BMI as an added way to monitor weight status.

Bone mineral density: the amount of bone tissue in a segment of bone, often measured to determine bone strength and predict fracture risk using T-scores and Z-scores. See also DEXA.

C

Cancer: a term used when there is uncontrolled and abnormal growth of cells in a specific part of the body, which can then sometimes spread (metastasize) through the bloodstream and lymphatic system to other parts of the body.

Cardiovascular disease (CVD): a general term for conditions affecting the heart (cardio) or blood vessels (vascular). It includes heart disease, coronary artery disease (CAD), and coronary or ischaemic heart disease (CHD) as well as peripheral vascular disease. CVD is one of the main causes of death and disability all over the world. The good news is that it is largely preventable with the help of a healthy lifestyle.

Carnitine: substance made in the muscle and liver tissue and found in certain foods, such as meat, poultry, fish and some dairy products. It is used by many cells in the body to make energy from fatty acids.

Cervix: neck or the narrow end of the womb (uterus) that leads into the vagina. A cervical or Pap smear is used to detect abnormal cells in the cervix to prevent and reduce the risk of developing cervical cancer.

Chemotherapy: treatment that uses drugs to stop the growth of cancer cells, either by killing the cells or by stopping them from dividing. These drugs may induce an early medical menopause for many women.

Cholesterol: a natural waxy fatty substance found in all cells of the body and in the blood. It is produced in the liver and is also in some of the foods we eat. Cholesterol is important to keep the cells in our bodies healthy. It is the substrate or base from which sex hormones, progesterone, oestrogen and testosterone are produced in the body through a complex pathway.

Chronic disease: a long-term condition or illness.

Circadian rhythm: biological changes that occur over an approximately 24-hour cycle as part of the body's internal clock. They are dependent in large part on environmental cues like light and darkness to help the brain regulate biological processes such as sleep/wake cycles and the release of hormones.

Clinical: concerned with or based on actual observation and treatment of disease in patients rather than experimentation or theory.

Cognition: or intellectual functioning is the use of conscious and unconscious mental processes by which knowledge and understanding are gained. For example, it includes thinking, remembering, recognizing and problem-solving.

Cognitive behavioural therapy (CBT): talking therapy that can help you manage your problems by changing the way you think and behave.

Combined oral contraceptive pill (COCP): hormonal contraception containing both oestrogen and progesterone.

Complementary and alternative medicine (CAM): treatments that are not usually part of conventional mainstream healthcare, including homeopathy, aromatherapy, meditation and acupuncture. A therapy is called 'complementary' when it is used in addition to conventional medicine, whereas it is called 'alternative' when it is used instead of conventional therapies.

Coriander: a herb, also known as cilantro.

C-reactive protein (CRP): plasma protein that rises in the blood when there is inflammation or infection. It can be identified by a simple blood test.

D

Dementia: an umbrella term for a range of progressive conditions that affect the brain. A gradual loss of memory and other intellectual abilities as a result of damage or disease in the brain beyond what is expected in normal cognitive ageing. Alzheimer's is the most common type of dementia.

Depression: a condition that is marked by a persistent sad, anxious or low mood that can last a long time or keep returning, affecting everyday life, often with feelings of hopelessness that affect eating, sleeping and other daily activities. Major depression can coexist alongside mood changes and other perimenopausal and menopausal symptoms.

DEXA: or dual-energy x-ray absorptiometry (DEXA) scan is the standard test used to measure bone mineral density, using a low dose of radiation. See also Bone mineral density.

Diabetes: a group of diseases which can cause a person's blood sugar level to become too high. There are many forms of diabetes. The most common ones are type 2 diabetes which responds very well to lifestyle management to treat the underlying cause of insulin resistance and type 1 diabetes when the body does not produce enough insulin.

Diabetes may cause a number of complications over time such as cardiovascular disease, blindness and kidney failure.

Disordered eating: variety of abnormal eating behaviours and body image concerns that, by themselves, do not warrant diagnosis of an eating disorder. Some of the most common types of disordered eating are dieting and restrictive eating.

E

Early menopause: when periods stop between the ages of 40 and 45.

Endocrine system: series of glands that produce hormones that work their effect on distant organs, controlling important functions such as reproduction, through a complex messenger system with feedback loops.

Endometrial ablation: A surgical procedure where the inner lining of the uterus or endometrium is removed to treat heavy periods.

Endometrial hyperplasia: condition in which the lining of the uterus grows too thick.

Endometriosis: a chronic condition when tissue similar to the lining of the uterus (endometrial lining) grows outside the womb (uterus), on the ovaries, fallopian tubes, bowel, bladder, back of the uterus and sometimes in scars and distant organs. Symptoms include heavy and/or painful periods, painful sex, infertility, bloating and chronic fatigue. It takes an average of 7–8 years to be diagnosed.

Endometrium: inner lining of the womb (uterus) or endometrial lining.

Endometrial or uterine cancer: refers to cancer of this lining.

Estrogen: see Oestrogen.

Evidence-based: the use of the best available scientific evidence from the most current academic research to make clinical decisions.

EVOO: extra virgin olive oil.

Excess weight: excess body fat.

F

Fasting blood sugar: test to determine how much glucose (sugar) is in a blood sample after an overnight fast.

Fibroids: smooth muscle growths that grow in and around the womb (uterus). These extremely common growths, also known as leiomyomas or myomas, are almost always benign (non-cancerous). Fibroids may cause no symptoms but can cause abnormal uterine bleeding, tummy swelling or fertility issues and should be investigated and treated if causing problems, even in the menopause.

Final menstrual period (FMP): the last or final menstrual period in a person's life.

Follicle-stimulating hormone (FSH): hormone made by the pituitary gland in the brain that helps an egg to mature and regulates the menstrual cycle. FSH levels rise in menopause.

Free sugars: includes all monosaccharides and disaccharides added to foods by the manufacturer, cook or consumer, plus sugars naturally present in honey, syrups and unsweetened fruit juices. Within this definition, lactose (milk sugar) when naturally present in milk and milk products and sugars contained within the cellular structure of foods (particularly fruits and vegetables) are excluded.

G

Genitourinary syndrome of menopause (GSM): includes menopausal symptoms and signs that affect both the vaginal area and the lower urinary tract due to low levels of the hormone oestrogen.

Gonadotropin-releasing hormone (GnRH): a hormone released by the hypothalamus, located in the brain, that regulates and releases hormones such as FSH and LH from the pituitary gland. Drugs similar to GnRH are sometimes prescribed to shrink fibroids, manage endometriosis, in breast cancer treatment or to control abnormal uterine bleeding.

H

Hormone replacement therapy (HRT, MHT, HT): the use of hormonal treatment prescribed by qualified health professionals during perimenopause and menopause to help relieve menopause symptoms such as hot flushes and mood swings, caused by oestrogen deficiency. The most common hormones used are oestrogen and progesterone, sometimes with the addition of testosterone. HRT is the same as MHT (menopausal hormone therapy) or HT (hormone therapy).

Hormones: chemical messengers that are released directly into the blood, which carries them to distant organs and tissues of the body to exert their functions.

Hot flush or hot flash: the sudden intense feeling of warmth, usually over the face, neck and chest, causing redness, rapid heartbeat and sweating and sometimes, feeling chilly afterwards. Night sweats are hot flushes that happen at night, and they may disrupt sleep. Although other medical conditions can cause them, hot flushes most commonly are due to menopause.

Human papillomavirus (HPV): a group of viruses responsible for the most common sexually transmitted infection (STI), affecting nearly all sexually active people at some point in their lives. Most people clear HPV on their own but HPV can cause abnormal changes in the cervix, vulva, vagina, penis, anus and other tissues when treatment may be needed.

Hypertension: abnormally high blood pressure.

Hypoactive sexual desire disorder: common in perimenopause and menopause with problems noted with sexual desire, sexual pain, arousal and orgasm.

Hypothalamic amenorrhoea (HA): a diagnosis of exclusion and said to occur when periods stop in the reproductive age due to hypothalamic dysfunction, often due to stress, excessive exercise and/or weight loss, known as functional HA.

Hysterectomy: surgical removal of the uterus and includes the cervix in most situations.

Hysteroscopy: a minimally invasive surgical procedure to examine the endometrial lining of the uterus. Small fibroids and uterine polyps are often removed with this technique and is also used to investigate abnormal bleeding, including post-menopausal bleeding.

I

Incontinence: can be urinary (stress or urge) or faecal and both may be seen in menopause. It is the involuntary loss of bladder or bowel control.

Infertility: often used interchangeably with subfertility, is a disease of the male or female reproductive system, defined by the WHO as the failure to achieve a pregnancy after 12 months or more of regular unprotected sexual intercourse. Approximately one in every six people of reproductive age worldwide experiences infertility in their lifetime.

Insomnia: defined as difficulty falling asleep, staying asleep, or waking early. Women are affected twice as much as men.

Insulin-like growth factor-1 (IGF-1): a hormone that, along with growth hormone, helps promote normal bone and tissue growth and development.

Insulin resistance: when cells in your body are unable to respond to the hormone insulin and therefore cannot take up glucose. This is the main cause of type 2 diabetes but occurs in a number of related conditions including PCOS.

Intrauterine device (IUD, IUCD, IUS): long-acting reversible contraceptive device and may contain either progesterone or copper. The intrauterine system (IUS) containing progesterone may also be used for managing heavy periods and as the progesterone arm of HRT.

Irritable bowel syndrome (IBS): common condition that affects the digestive system. It causes symptoms such as stomach cramps, bloating, diarrhoea and constipation.

Isoflavones: contain phytoestrogens which are naturally occurring oestrogen-like compounds found in soya beans, soya products and red clover.

L

LGBTQIA+: lesbian, gay, bisexual, transgender, queer (or sometimes questioning), intersex, asexual, and others. The 'plus' represents other sexual identities, including pansexual and two-spirit.

Libido: sexual desire.

Lifestyle medicine (LM): as defined by the American College of Lifestyle Medicine (ACLM), the use of evidence-based, lifestyle, therapeutic interventions – including a whole-food, plant-predominant eating pattern, regular physical activity, restorative sleep, stress management, avoidance of risky substances, and positive social connection – as a primary modality, delivered by clinicians trained in these modalities, to prevent, treat and often reverse disease.

Lignans: type of naturally occurring plant oestrogens, for example in flaxseed.

Local vaginal oestrogen: can be used as a ring, cream or pessary. This form of treatment can be used indefinitely in most women safely to manage symptoms of GSM, including vaginal dryness.

Luteinizing hormone (LH): a hormone made in the pituitary gland that helps an egg to be released from the ovary.

M

Macronutrients: nutrients that provide most of the energy, or fuel, the human body needs to function properly. Macronutrients include proteins, carbohydrates and fats. These nutrients provide the calories (energy) in your diet.

Mammogram: breast screening method using X-rays to detect abnormal growths or changes in the breast tissue. Ultrasound and MRI of the breast are other less commonly used screening methods.

Medical menopause: when menopause is induced as a result of certain drugs such as chemotherapy or GnRH medications or radiotherapy treatment. Symptoms of menopause may start abruptly.

Menarche: the first menstrual period.

Menopausal or post-menopausal: terms used for the time frame after the 12 months of a woman completely stopping her menstrual cycles.

Menopausal hormone therapy (MHT): see Hormone replacement therapy (HRT).

Menopause: the final or last menstrual period a woman will ever have. It is a diagnosis made in retrospect, as it is defined as the absence of periods for more than 12 months. This is sometimes also known as natural or spontaneous menopause unlike induced medical or surgical menopause.

Menopause transition: see perimenopause.

Menstrual cycle: changes that occur over the course of 25–35 days during the reproductive years in a menstruating person's life. The endometrial lining thickens in preparation for accepting a fertilized egg. If fertilization of the egg with a sperm does not occur, the lining is shed, causing a bleed, which is called a period (menstruation).

Menstruation: or a period is that part of the menstrual cycle that occurs as vaginal bleeding every month (25–35 days' interval) for a few days (1–7 days' duration). A period consists of a discharge of blood, secretions and tissue debris shed by the uterus. Heavy or painful or missing periods should not be ignored, especially if lasting more than three months and earlier, if there are any concerns.

Metabolic syndrome: combination of problems that can lead to type 2 diabetes and heart disease. These problems include high blood pressure, having excess weight or having too much fat around your waist, higher-than-normal blood sugar level, lower-than-normal levels of 'good' cholesterol, and high levels of fats in the blood (triglycerides).

Micronutrients: include vitamins and minerals, as well as compounds like phytonutrients (plant nutrients) that play a vital role in optimal health. Micronutrients are only needed in tiny amounts. Eating a varied diet, rich in colourful fruits and vegetables, is the best way to get all the necessary micronutrients.

Magnetic resonance imaging (MRI): an imaging technique that allows the soft tissues of the body to be seen. An MRI of the pelvis may be requested as part of the investigations for fibroids, endometriosis, adenomyosis and cancers such as endometrial cancer.

Minimally processed: foods that are in their natural or nearly natural state, with inedible parts removed and retaining most of the nutrients.

O

Obesity: state characterized by excessive body fat.

Oestrogen: the main female sex hormone, influencing the growth and maintaining the health of female reproductive organs. There are three major naturally occurring oestrogens: oestrone (E1), oestradiol (E2) and oestriol (E3). Oestradiol is the most abundant in the pre-menopausal phase of life. Oestrogen levels gradually fall in menopause unless menopause is medically or surgically induced, when levels can drop abruptly.

Osteoarthritis (OA): the most common form of joint disease, causing joints to become painful and stiff, often with swelling. This condition increases with the 'wear and tear' of ageing, particularly in women.

Osteopenia: the stage before osteoporosis, diagnosed on a bone density scan showing reduced bone density. Osteopenia does not always lead to osteoporosis.

Osteoporosis: a disease when bones become fragile and are at higher risk for fractures, often with little or no trauma. Bone loss accelerates during the first few years after menopause, which is related to the drop in oestrogen levels.

Ovary: there are usually two reproductive glands or ovaries, one on either side of the uterus within the pelvis, producing eggs and hormones for menstruation and pregnancy. The ovaries are the main source of oestrogen, progesterone and testosterone hormones before menopause.

Ovulation: the release of one or more eggs from the ovary in response to hormones.

Oxidative stress: imbalance between free radicals and antioxidants in your body.

P

Pelvic examination: a clinical examination of the vulva, vagina, cervix, uterus and ovaries, which can provide useful information in some situations. An instrument called a vaginal speculum is inserted into the vagina and a Pap test (cervical smear), swabs and biopsies may be done during this exam. You can decline an internal pelvic examination, especially if you have never had penetrative vaginal sex, and you can request a chaperone.

Pelvis: the lower part of the abdomen, located between the hip bones.

Perimenopause or menopause in transition: the lead up to menopause. Perimenopause typically lasts for four years, but may last 2–8 years.

Period: see Menstruation.

Phytoestrogens: plant oestrogens including isoflavones and lignans. Phytoestrogens are found in several different types of food such as soya, grains, beans, and some fruits and vegetables.

Placebo: typically an inactive substance, may be used in controlled trials to test the efficacy of another substance (such as a drug).

Polycystic ovary syndrome/polycystic ovarian syndrome (PCOS): sometimes known as PCOD (polycystic ovarian disorder) is an endocrine disorder whereby polycystic ovaries are one of an array of possible symptoms caused by an underlying hormone imbalance.

Polyphenols: compounds naturally found in plants that have antioxidant and anti-inflammatory properties.

Prediabetes: condition in which blood sugar is high, but not high enough to be diagnosed as type 2 diabetes.

Premature ovarian failure (POF) (premature menopause): a condition that causes the ovaries to stop working before age 40. POI is the preferred term.

Premature ovarian insufficiency (POI): a condition that causes the ovaries to stop working before age 40. HRT is indicated for most people with POI.

Premenstrual syndrome (PMS): name for the symptoms women can experience in the weeks before their period. These include mood swings, tender breasts, food cravings, fatigue, irritability and depression.

Progestogens: natural or synthetic hormones that have similar actions to the hormone progesterone that circulates in a woman's body.

Progesterone: a hormone released by the ovary. It has an important role in the menstrual cycle and is vital in maintaining the early stages of pregnancy.

Prolactin: hormone made by the pituitary gland, a small gland at the base of the brain. It causes the breasts to grow and make milk during pregnancy and after birth.

Prolapse: or uterovaginal or pelvic organ prolapse is the slipping of a body part from its usual position (for example, uterus or bladder or rectal prolapse, if the ligaments holding it in place become stretched).

R

Reproductive age: from the start of your first period until menopause is reached.

S

SERM: or selective oestrogen receptor modulator can both mimic and block the effects of oestrogen in various tissues. These hormones have beneficial oestrogen effects in certain areas of the body and block unwanted oestrogen effects in other parts of the body.

SSRIs and SNRIs: or selective serotonin reuptake inhibitors (SSRIs) block the reabsorption (reuptake) of the neurotransmitter serotonin in the brain and are the most widely used antidepressant. Serotonin-noradrenaline reuptake inhibitors (SNRIs) are another group of antidepressants. Both may be used in menopause.

Surgical menopause: when menopause is induced from surgical removal of both of the ovaries (bilateral oophorectomy) for medical reasons. Symptoms are often more intense and start abruptly in this situation.

T

Testosterone: see Androgen. In women, increased levels of testosterone can lead to acne and hirsutism. Low levels of testosterone in women may contribute to loss of libido.

Transdermal: absorbed through the skin as with some oestrogen patches, creams or gels.

U

Ultraprocessed or highly processed: foods with many added ingredients such as sugar, salt, fat, and artificial colours or preservatives. Ultra-processed foods are made mostly from substances extracted from foods, such as fats, starches, added sugars and hydrogenated fats.

Ultrasound scan: a pelvic ultrasound or sonogram uses high frequency sound waves to produce an electronic image of the organs of the pelvis. A transvaginal ultrasound is performed via the vagina and can give more information.

Uterus: womb.

V

Vagina: a tube-like structure surrounded by muscles. The vagina leads from the cervix and uterus to the outside of the body.

Vasomotor symptoms: such as hot flushes and night sweats experienced in perimenopause and menopause.

Vulva: external female genital area.

Vulvodynia: pain in the vulva, usually described as a burning, stinging or irritating feeling.

W

WHO: World Health Organization – a part of the United Nations that deals with major health issues around the world.

Women's Health Initiative (WHI): large research trials established by the National Institutes of Health in 1991 in the USA to investigate strategies for the prevention and control of common chronic diseases in post-menopausal women. Most media reports refer to oral hormone therapy initiated in older women (past perimenopause) to determine its relationship to cardiovascular disease, stroke, breast cancer, osteoporosis, colon cancer, and other conditions.

Popular diet patterns

Plant-based: consisting or made completely of plants, or mainly of plants.

Vegetarianism: a diet pattern that excludes meat, poultry and fish but sometimes includes eggs and dairy.

Veganism: an ethical lifestyle that excludes all animal-derived food from the diet, including meat, poultry, fish, eggs, dairy and honey.

Whole-food, plant-based diet: consists of all whole or minimally processed fruit, vegetables, whole grains, legumes, nuts and seeds, herbs and spices. It excludes all animal products, including red meat, poultry, fish, eggs and dairy products. This diet pattern minimizes the consumption of added salt, oil and sugar.

Acknowledgements

A couple of years ago, if someone had said I would be writing my second book so soon after my first one, I would not have believed them. Writing my first book with Rohini was such a joyful process, despite the many moments of doubt, that I was eager to get back to writing. The positive response for *Living PCOS Free* has been so encouraging, with people reaching out to say how helpful they have found the book.

My own encounter with a much earlier menopause more than a couple of decades ago at the age of 38 was not straightforward. I would have loved a book like *Finding Me in Menopause* to help me navigate the myths and confusion that were out there. Despite ample scientific evidence, health professionals and women still remain unsure about the power of nutrition and lifestyle in improving health, particularly in perimenopause and menopause. My hope with the book is to clearly explain the benefits, using the latest available research.

I am grateful to so many people for making this book happen but most of all to you, my dear reader.

Victoria Roddam, my publisher at Hodder & Stoughton, reached out to me to write a book on menopause. Victoria, your belief in me has been empowering. This was a book I already had in me but you managed to tease it out of me in record time. Your suggestions and edits have been invaluable. You knew when to reign me in and when to allow me to write what I wanted to convey. Not imposing a rigid word limit meant I could discuss so many issues dear to my heart. I can't thank you enough. Your team have been just brilliant.

A huge hooray and thank you to my friends Dave and Steve Flynn of The Happy Pear for collaborating with me on The Happy Menopause Course. Your recipes are going to be so well received. You guys are the best.

To my soulmate of 43 years, Rajiv. Your smooth handling of the running of the house, feeding me amazing plant-based meals, walking our dogs twice a day to relieve me of my duty when the deadline was looming have not gone unnoticed. People are going to find your chapter on bone health in menopause very helpful and easy to understand. They will enjoy your delicious recipe. Thank you. I love you.

To our older daughter, Rohini. You are my constant editor, wise beyond your years. Your input into the entire book with your fabulous suggestions and attention to detail and critique are the reasons why *Finding Me in Menopause* has been so enjoyable to write. I marvel at your patience when I send you messages at all hours of the day, refusing to get annoyed, even with the most obvious query. Your chapter on ensuring adequate protein as we get older will no doubt help many women as it has helped me. The tips on bloating and the nutritious chia seed recipe will be a great hit in the book.

A very big thank you to our younger daughter, Naina, for always inspiring me to be a better person. You took out precious time from your busy day job, making the book a much better read with your invaluable comments. I love you both very much.

To my friends, Daisy, Prayna and Michelle, for your positive encouragement after reading my first draft so promptly. I would also like to acknowledge my family and friends, including my son-in-law, Siddhant, my nieces, Vaidehi and Anisha Samat, my book club and golf group friends for their support.

To our adorable dogs, Kappu and Tippu. Your loyalty and love never fail to amaze me.

I have dedicated this book to my amazing parents, Vimala and Venkataraman, and my wonderful parents-in-law, Manorama and Atmaram. Your support meant the world to me. You may be no more but you are all always in my heart.

Finally, I want to express my gratitude to my patients. I have learnt from each and every one of you. Thank you.

About the experts

Dr Nitu Bajekal MD FRCOG ObGyn Dip IBLM

Dr Nitu Bajekal, MD is a Senior Consultant Obstetrician and Gynaecologist in London, UK, with nearly 40 years of clinical experience in women's health. Her special interests include lifestyle medicine, menopause, PCOS, endometriosis, period problems, complex vulval problems and medical education. She is a keyhole surgeon with experience in laparoscopic procedures including robotics.

She is a Fellow of the Royal College and recipient of the Indian President's Gold Medal.

Dr Bajekal is one of the first board-certified Lifestyle Medicine Physicians in the UK. She has written the women's health module for the first UK plant-based nutrition course at Winchester University. She has co-authored the women's health chapter for an academic book for health professionals (*Plant-Based Nutrition in Clinical Practice*, Hammersmith Books, September 2022).

She has lectured on the Holistic Holiday at Sea (HHAS) programme on menopause, PCOS and women's health issues.

Dr Bajekal is passionate about educating women, providing reliable medical and lifestyle information for the general public, doctors, workplaces and schools. She runs a voluntary service set up to educate, energize and empower schoolgirls and women to make lifestyle choices to help improve their own and their families' health.

Dr Bajekal is the co-author of *Living PCOS Free*, a practical guide to managing polycystic ovary syndrome (PCOS) with proven lifestyle approaches alongside Western medicine. She has written this book with her daughter, Rohini Bajekal. It is available worldwide via all major book outlets and Amazon (Hammersmith Health Books, April 2022).

Her latest work involves leading a menopause course to help women through the perimenopause and menopause, busting myths, discussing hormone therapy and the importance of lifestyle in the successful management of menopause (The Happy Menopause Course, October 2022) in collaboration with The Happy Pear.

Read more about her work, profile, podcasts and recipes on her website, with over 50 free women's health information leaflets and resources: https://nitubajekal.com/

Follow her on Instagram @drnitubajekal and TikTok where she shares health tips, recipes and more.

Dr Rajiv Bajekal MS, FRCS Orth. MCh Orth. Dip IBLM

Dr Rajiv Bajekal is a Consultant Spinal Surgeon practising in London, United Kingdom. He has nearly 40 years of clinical experience in orthopaedics and subsequently specialized in spinal surgery. His surgical practice is mainly in the lumbar spine with a keen interest in managing sciatica, low back pain, spinal stenosis, osteoporotic fractures and infections. He is particularly keen to find simple and often non-surgical solutions for patients in severe pain and practises lifestyle medicine to look at problems more holistically rather than just the presenting problem.

Dr Bajekal is a senior examiner for the FRCS Trauma and Orthopaedic Examination and lectures widely both nationally and internationally for general practitioners and is part of a group called Total Orthopaedics which provides high-quality patient-focused care. He is also a board-certified Lifestyle Medicine Practitioner who has personally experienced the healing benefits of a whole-food plant-based diet. Dr Bajekal has since become a passionate advocate for lifestyle medicine with his patients and has written a module and lectured on the UK's first plant-based nutrition course on bone health and osteoporosis conducted by Winchester University. He has also co-written a chapter on bone health for an academic book for health professionals titled *Plant-Based Nutrition in Clinical Practice* (September 2022).

He is passionate about teaching and lecturing, often making difficult areas of spinal surgery easy to understand.

For more information visit www.rajivbajekal.com and follow him on Instagram @drrajivbajekal

Rohini Bajekal MA Oxon MSc Dip IBLM

Rohini Bajekal is a nutritionist and board-certified Lifestyle Medicine professional. Prior to becoming a nutritionist, she studied theology at Oxford University. Having previously worked in India and Singapore, Rohini is now based in London and provides evidence-based nutrition and lifestyle advice to her clients around the world.

An avid recipe developer, Rohini is passionate about making delicious and nourishing plant-based meals. In her spare time, she volunteers as a cookery teacher at Made in Hackney, the UK's only plant-based cookery school and charity. Rohini leads communications at Plant-Based Health Professionals UK and is part of the Dietitian and Nutritionist Advisory Committee at Diet ID.

Together with her mother, Dr Nitu Bajekal, ObGyn, Rohini co-authored *Living PCOS Free: How to Regain Your Hormonal Health with Polycystic Ovary Syndrome*. Rohini has personal experience of polycystic ovary syndrome (PCOS). She also wrote the chapter on lifestyle medicine for the book *How to Go Plant-Based: A Definitive Guide for You and Your Family* by Ella Mills, founder of Deliciously Ella.

Subscribe to Rohini's free monthly newsletter and find out about her work at www.rohinibajekal.com. You can also follow her on Instagram @rohinibajekal for recipes and daily tips on plant-based living.

Index